When a Loved One at Home has Dementia:

A Family Member's Guide to Caring for a Loved One

By: Dr. Debbie Sue Francis

ISBN-10: 1477402268
EAN-13: 9781477402269

For my Beloved Jim,
and my mentor Lara

Table of Contents

5. Aphasia and Other Language Deficits (with clinical case examples)

6. How to Communicate with Your Loved One Who Has a Language Deficit (with clinical case examples) 69

7. Managing Your Loved One's Problem Behaviors (with clinical case examples) 79

1. What Is Dementia?

Dementia is a term used to describe a constellation of symptoms, rather than a specific disease. Dementia, as a nonspecific illness syndrome, can be diagnosed when a group of intellectual and social abilities are effected severely enough to interfere with daily functioning. When dementia is diagnosed, the cognitive areas affected can include memory, attention, language, and problem solving. These symptoms usually need to be present at least six months before the diagnosis of dementia can be made.

Dementia can be caused by many conditions. Some of the most common forms of dementia are Alzheimer's disease, vascular dementia, frontotemporal dementia, semantic dementia, and dementia with lewy bodies. It is possible for a patient to exhibit more than one dementing process at the same time.

Dementia is a condition usually associated with the elderly population, age sixty-five and older, but young adults can also experience dementia. It is rare to develop dementia as a young adult without other risk factors such as alcohol and drug abuse, brain injury, other neurological diseases, psychiatric illness, or other metabolic disturbances.

Memory loss is a prominent symptom of dementia, but memory loss alone doesn't mean you have dementia. In order to receive a diagnosis of dementia, the patient must suffer impairments in at least two brain functions, such as memory loss and impaired judgment or language. Some causes of dementia are treatable and even reversible, while some causes of dementia do not respond to treatment.

The etiology or cause of dementia determines its symptoms; however, general symptoms include: memory impairment, impaired communication, inability to learn or remember new information, impaired executive functioning, difficulty with coordination, personality and mood changes, inability to reason, inappropriate behavior, paranoia and hallucination, agitation and violence. Most patients do not present with all of these symptoms and each patient's symptom presentation is uniquely different.

Dementia's symptomology varies slightly depending on the cause; however, symptom overlap prevents diagnosis by symptomology alone of the dementia type. Therefore, only a qualified medical doctor can diagnose the types of dementia from which a Patient suffers.

The ways that dementias are classified vary by etiology (causes and origins) and by what they have in common. Progressive dementias are a class of dementias categorized by how and what part of the brain is affected or by how the dementias worsen. Reversible dementias are a class of dementias categorized by being reversible with treatment, such as those caused by a reaction to medications.

Progressive Dementias

Alzheimer's Disease

In the elderly population, Alzheimer's disease is one of the most common causes of dementia. Symptoms usually appear after age sixty, but in young adults, early-onset forms of the disease can occur. With Alzheimer's disease, there are two types of damage to the brain cells. These include plaques and tangles. One is normally harmless proteins called beta-amyloid; these are plaques. The other is fibrous tangles made up of an abnormal protein called tau protein. The progression of Alzheimer's disease is usually a gradual onset with a slow progression—over seven to ten years. Eventually, the cognitive functions of the brain no longer work properly, resulting in severe impairment to memory, movement, language, judgment, behavior, and abstract thinking (Alzheimer's Disease Education, 2012; Dementia Guide, 2011; Mayo Clinic, 2010; National Institute on Aging, 2011).

Lewy Body Dementia

Dementia with lewy bodies is one of the most common types of dementia in the elderly population. Lewy bodies are proteins abnormally formed in the brains of people with lewy body dementia, Alzheimer's disease, and Parkinson's disease. Lewy body dementia includes symptoms that are similar to Alzheimer's disease, with intermittent symptoms between alternating stages of confusion and clear thinking, visual hallucinations, and Parkinson's signs such as tremor and rigidity. Often with lewy body dementia, the patient will experience REM sleep behavior disorder that involves acting out dreams, which can involve kicking violently while sleeping (Alzheimer's Disease Education, 2012; Dementia Guide, 2011; Mayo Clinic, 2010; National Institute on Aging, 2011).

Vascular Dementia

Vascular dementia is a common type of dementia, almost as common as Alzheimer's disease. Vascular dementia is caused by damage to the brain resulting from problems with the arteries connected to the brain or heart. It has sudden onset, often after a stroke, and may occur in people with high blood pressure, or after a heart attack. Other risk factors for vascular dementia include infection of a heart valve or a buildup of amyloid protein in the brain's blood vessels that sometimes causes "bleeding" strokes.

There are several variations of vascular dementia with significant differences in their symptoms. In general, vascular dementia is more common in the elderly and often co-occurs with Alzheimer's disease. Some types affect only one side of the body, and some types cause cognitive impairment and personality changes. Some types of vascular dementia are progressive and some types respond to treatment (Alzheimer's Disease Education, 2012; Dementia Guide, 2011; Mayo Clinic, 2010; National Institute on Aging, 2011).

Frontotemporal Dementia

Frontotemporal dementia occurs in young adults and the elderly; it affects young adults more often than other dementias. The frontal and temporal lobes of the brain are associated with personality, executive function, decision making, and language. Frontotemporal dementia is a group of dementias characterized by a process of neuron degeneration in this area of the brain. Impairment in the frontal lobe region of the brain can result in socially inappropriate behaviors, language impairment, difficulty thinking, and mental rigidity. Little is known about the cause of frontotemporal dementia, although in some cases this dementia is related to certain genetic mutations (Alzheimer's Disease Education, 2012; Dementia Guide, 2011; Mayo Clinic, 2010; National Institute on Aging, 2011).

Other Disorders Linked to Dementia

Huntington's Disease

Huntington's disease is an inherited condition that causes degeneration of the nerve cells in the spinal cord. The onset of symptoms usually begins in early to mid-adulthood, around the late thirties. In the beginning, symptoms may include mild personality changes such as anxiety and depression. The symptoms eventually progress into severe dementia including difficulty with walking and other movement (Alzheimer's Disease Education,

2012; Dementia Guide, 2011; Mayo Clinic, 2010; National Institute on Aging, 2011).

Dementia Pugilistica

Dementia pugilistica or *boxer's dementia* is caused by chronic, repetitive head trauma. The symptoms vary according to the part of the brain that has been injured and range from memory problems, poor coordination, and impaired speech, to tremors, slow movement, and muscle stiffness. Symptoms may not appear until many years post-trauma. A single, acute head injury can cause post-traumatic dementia, which is much like dementia pugilistica, but in this case, the memory loss can be permanent (Alzheimer's Disease Education, 2012; Dementia Guide, 2011; Mayo Clinic, 2010; National Institute on Aging, 2011).

HIV-Associated Dementia

Infection with the human immunodeficiency virus (HIV) can cause degeneration of neurons and cortical structures, resulting in symptomology similar to other dementias: for example, memory loss, social withdrawal, difficulty with concentration, and impaired motor function (Alzheimer's Disease Education, 2012; Dementia Guide, 2011; Mayo Clinic, 2010; National Institute on Aging, 2011).

Creutzfeldt-Jakob Disease

This type of dementia is rare and usually fatal, and the cause is unknown; it often occurs in the elderly population rather than in young adulthood. Heredity and exposure to diseased brain or nervous system tissue can be a risk factor. Signs and symptoms initially include problems with coordination and balance, vision difficulties, personality changes, and impaired memory, cognition, judgment, and thinking. Cognitive impairment becomes more severe as the illness progresses. The end stage of this illness often includes blindness, pneumonia, and other infections (Alzheimer's Disease Education, 2012; Dementia Guide, 2011; Mayo Clinic, 2010; National Institute on Aging, 2011).

Secondary Dementias

Other disorders can sometimes result in symptoms of dementia; for example, people with Parkinson's are likely to develop symptoms of dementia as their disease progresses. Chronic inflammatory conditions of the brain, such as multiple sclerosis and systematic lupus, may affect cognition in the long term. Currently, the relationship between these disorders and dementia isn't completely understood (Alzheimer's Disease Education, 2012; Dementia Guide, 2011; Mayo Clinic, 2010; National Institute on Aging, 2011).

Causes of Dementia That Can Be Reversed

Infectious and Immune Disorders

Dementia can occur when your body attempts to fight disease or infections, or as a consequence of fever. For example, conditions like multiple sclerosis can result from the immune system's defense of the body's nerve cells and cause dementia. Other conditions can cause dementia, like meningitis and encephalitis, untreated syphilis, Lyme disease, and conditions such as leukemia that cause a completely compromised immune system. (Alzheimer's Disease Education, 2012; Dementia Guide, 2011; Mayo Clinic, 2010; National Institute on Aging, 2011).

Metabolic Problems and Endocrine Abnormalities

Several risk factors can contribute to the vulnerability to developing symptoms, including thyroid problems, too little sugar in the bloodstream (hypoglycemia), calcium abnormalities, and an impaired ability to absorb vitamin B_{12} (Alzheimer's Disease Education, 2012; Dementia Guide, 2011; Mayo Clinic, 2010; National Institute on Aging, 2011).

Nutritional Deficiencies

Nutritional risk factors that can contribute to vulnerability to developing symptoms of dementia include dehydration, not having enough thiamine (vitamin B_1), vitamins B_6 and B_{12} deficiencies (Alzheimer's Disease Education, 2012; Dementia Guide, 2011; Mayo Clinic, 2010; National Institute on Aging, 2011).

Reactions to Medications

Reactions to medications may cause dementia symptoms in reaction to several different medications or one medication. These reactions can be to prescription medication or over-the-counter medications (Alzheimer's Disease Education, 2012; Dementia Guide, 2011; Mayo Clinic, 2010; National Institute on Aging, 2011).

Subdural Hematomas

Subdural hematoma is a condition in which bleeding occurs between the brain's outer surface and the brain itself. Subdural hematoma can be a consequence of several different events (Alzheimer's Disease Education, 2012; Dementia Guide, 2011; Mayo Clinic, 2010; National Institute on Aging, 2011).

Poisoning

Environmental teratogen can cause dementia; for example, from lead or other poisons like pesticides. Dementia can be a result from long-term, chronic substance abuse like alcohol, known as Korsokoff Syndrome . When dementia is a result of poisoning, it might be possible to treat the symptoms, and the symptoms might go away after the exposure to the substance is discontinued (Alzheimer's Disease Education, 2012; Dementia Guide, 2011; Mayo Clinic, 2010; National Institute on Aging, 2011).

Brain Tumors

Dementia symptoms can be the consequence of a brain tumor and the subsequent damage caused to the cortical structures. When a brain tumor is the cause of dementia, the condition might or might not respond to treatment (Alzheimer's Disease Education, 2012; Dementia Guide, 2011; Mayo Clinic, 2010; National Institute on Aging, 2011).

Anoxia

Caused by severe oxygen depletion to vital cortical structures and other vital tissue, the condition anoxia/hypoxia occurs. Causes range from myocardial infarction, asthma, and environmental poisoning, to high altitude. Depending of the severity of the hypoxia, the recovery time varies as does the symptomology (Alzheimer's Disease Education, 2012; Dementia Guide, 2011; Mayo Clinic, 2010; National Institute on Aging, 2011).

Heart and Lung Problems

Chronic heart or lung problems may deprive the brain of oxygen, which can result in dementia symptoms. Symptomology may vary depending on the individual conditions. (Alzheimer's Disease Education, 2012; Dementia Guide, 2011; Mayo Clinic, 2010; National Institute on Aging, 2011)

Risk Factors That Can't Be Changed

Age

The risk of developing dementia correlates positively with age; however, several types of dementia can develop as early-onset dementia and age, with these types of dementia, is not a risk factor. Healthy aging itself does not carry with it any symptomology of any form of dementia. (Alzheimer's Disease Education, 2012; Dementia Guide, 2011; Mayo Clinic, 2010; National Institute on Aging, 2011).

Family History

Hereditary factors can increase your risk of developing dementias. When a family history of dementia exists, a greater likelihood of developing dementia also exists. However, many people who have family histories that include dementia never develop dementia and likewise, many people who do *not* have family histories that include dementia, do in fact develop dementia. There is genetic testing available to determine whether or not you have certain types of genetic mutations that might develop into dementia but only for specific disorders where the specific types of mutations are known; for example, Huntington 's disease. Many of the mutations responsible for the diseases that cause dementia symptoms are not known and are therefore not available for testing (Alzheimer's Disease Education, 2012;Dementia Guide, 2011; Mayo Clinic, 2010; National Institute on Aging, 2011).

Down Syndrome

People born with Down syndrome will probably develop dementia symptoms similar to Alzheimer's disease by the time they are young adults (Alzheimer's Disease Education, 2012;Dementia Guide, 2011; Mayo Clinic, 2010; National Institute on Aging, 2011).

Risk Factors That Can Be Changed

Although there is still much that is unknown about the causes and risk factors related to many forms of dementia, while working toward reducing your risk of developing dementia, you can do several things to control the following factors.

Alcohol Use

Over consumption of alcoholic beverages can contribute to the risk of developing dementia symptoms. Some studies have shown, however, that moderate alcohol consumption can be a health benefit. One glass of red wine per day for women and two glasses of red wine per day for men may have health benefits (Alzheimer's Disease Education, 2012;Dementia Guide, 2011; Mayo Clinic, 2010; National Institute on Aging, 2011).

Atherosclerosis

When fatty substances build up inside the artery walls, the risk for developing vascular dementia becomes significant, as does the risk for heart disease and stroke. Studies have shown possible connections to arthrosclerosis and Alzheimer's disease (Alzheimer's Disease Education, 2012; Dementia Guide, 2011; Mayo Clinic, 2010; National Institute on Aging, 2011).

Blood Pressure

Hypertension (high blood pressure) as well as hypotension (low blood pressure) is a significant risk factor for several different types of dementias (Alzheimer's Disease Education, 2012; Dementia Guide, 2011; Mayo Clinic, 2010; National Institute on Aging, 2011).

Cholesterol

Risk factors for some types of dementia, including Alzheimer's disease, include maintaining high levels of LDL ("bad" cholesterol); maintaining higher levels of HDL ("good" cholesterol) might serve as a protective factor (Alzheimer's Disease Education, 2012; Dementia Guide, 2011; Mayo Clinic, 2010; National Institute on Aging, 2011).

Depression

Increased likelihood of developing dementia symptoms is associated with those who are diagnosed with symptoms of depression as adults. This risk factor does not seem to be as prevalent for women as it does for men when correlating with development of dementia symptomology (Alzheimer's Disease Education, 2012; Dementia Guide, 2011; Mayo Clinic, 2010; National Institute on Aging, 2011).

Diabetes

A diagnosis of diabetes, especially type 2 diabetes, increases the likelihood of developing several different types of dementia symptoms (Alzheimer's Disease Education, 2012;Dementia Guide, 2011; Mayo Clinic, 2010; National Institute on Aging, 2011).

High Estrogen Levels

Some studies have associated high combined levels of estrogen in women as a risk factor for developing dementia (Alzheimer's Disease Education, 2012; Dementia Guide, 2011; Mayo Clinic, 2010; National Institute on Aging, 2011).

Homocysteine Blood Levels

Some studies have associated elevated blood levels of homocysteine, a type of amino acid produced by your body, as a risk factor for developing several types of dementia (Alzheimer's Disease Education, 2012; Dementia Guide, 2011; Mayo Clinic, 2010; National Institute on Aging, 2011).

Smoking

Smoking is probably a significant risk factor in the development of several types of dementia because of the severe structural damage it causes to your vascular system, lungs, and neural tissue (Alzheimer's Disease Education, 2012; Dementia Guide, 2011; Mayo Clinic, 2010; National Institute on Aging, 2011).

2. Symptoms of Dementia

Progression of dementia can be categorized in three stages and is measured by the symptoms the person experiences. Usually, when someone is in the early stage of dementia, they are experiencing mild symptoms, and you or your loved one might not realize they are ill until they progress to a later stage. You may notice some unusual behaviors like irritability or forgetfulness, but the person might be able to employ some strategies like using detailed lists or using extra writing on their calendar to help them manage their daily activities. It might not be until the symptoms become more severe that you realize your loved one has dementia.

Early Stage Symptoms (Mild Dementia)

In the beginning, as your loved one first starts to show signs of dementia, you will notice things they might not notice. If you try to convince them of something they are sure is not happening, then they might become suspicious or frightened of you and, compounded by their experiencing dementia symptoms, this can be confusing for them.

Some of the symptoms of dementia occur on a continuum of normal human experiences. We all forget where we put our eyeglasses from time to time, but we eventually remember where we left them. We might not be able to recall someone's name or a telephone number we often use. This is normal. Someone with dementia experiences a constellation of symptoms, not just one or two things that happen once or twice. In other words, in addition to forgetting where they left their eyeglasses, and an important telephone number, they will also exhibit behavior problems, problems with executive functioning, disturbance with mood, and personality changes.

The following list includes several common symptoms many people with dementia might exhibit with descriptions of how each symptom might manifest itself in a daily experience:

Memory Loss

Normal memory vs. memory loss in dementia: when people with depression or normal memory loss forget where they put their keys or forget someone's name, they can remember this information with the help of cues, or in time, this information will come back to them. When people with dementia forget where they put something or forget someone's name, they usually never recall this information, even with the assistance of cues. No matter how long they think about it, the information is usually gone forever.

You might begin to experience your loved one as confused even before they realize they are experiencing memory loss. You may notice them asking the same question over and over, forgetting about important appointments, unable to remember familiar places or the names of loved ones. It is not uncommon for people to try to hide their experience or even to become defensive and try to prevent others from finding out they are having this frightening experience. Because your loved one might not understand what is happening to them, they can become frustrated and even hostile to prevent others from knowing they are in this unfamiliar world.

Difficulty Planning/Becoming Disorganized

Some people may begin to have difficulty with their daily routines. They may show difficulty with the ability to follow through with things like making a shopping list, then going to the grocery store, then putting the groceries away, then using the food to prepare a meal, and then cleaning up after themselves, washing the dishes and putting them away. It might appear as though they have just lost interest in what they have begun doing or like they have become frustrated with their task and gotten overwhelmed and therefore failed to complete their task.

Some people have difficulty driving to familiar places and can get lost in a neighborhood where they have lived for many years. They might have difficulty working with numbers and managing their checkbook or their household budget. Household chores might become unmanageable, and you might notice a difference in the way their home is kept. Someone who has always been very tidy and kept a clean house might begin to appear unkempt or disorganized at home and with their appearance.

Personal Hygiene

Personal hygiene may become difficult for some people to manage. Some people forget to bathe or might become frightened to bathe because of confusion and a feeling of vulnerability in the bathroom. Oral hygiene can suffer if the person forgets when they last brushed their teeth. Confusion about carrying out the task can be a barrier. Changing clothing from daytime attire to nighttime attire might be confusing and sometimes, days might pass before they change clothes at all. It is not uncommon for a person who is suffering from dementia to wear the same clothing for many days without noticing their clothing has become dirty. It can be a challenge to encourage a loved one to change clothing daily, because they might not realize they have been wearing the same clothing for so long.

Time and Place Confusion

Your loved one may become confused about events that will happen in the future or that happened in the past because tracking a time line can become difficult. They might have difficulty understanding time or the day of the week, seasons, or months. They might have difficulty with increments of time like "a few minutes," or "an hour." This can lead to confusion about where they are or how they got there because sometimes they can understand only what is going on this very minute.

Changes in Vision

For some people with dementia, vision can present a problem. They might have difficulty distinguishing colors or distance. Judging how fast something is moving can be difficult, which can lead to bumping into objects or falling. Sometimes, they might mistake inanimate objects for people, or they might think their own reflection in a mirror is another person and they might try to carry on a conversation with their reflection.

Difficulty Eating

Overeating or neglecting to eat can be a challenge for people suffering from dementia. Eating objects that are not edible can also be a problem for people with dementia. Loss of taste or ability to smell food along with the inability to remember to eat can present difficulty when trying to get a loved one to continue to eat regularly. Using a routine where meals are a fun and celebrated part of the day can be helpful as well as trying to incorporate your loved one's favorite foods and recipes.

Language/Self-Expression/ Communication

Your loved one may have difficulty following a conversation or being able to contribute in a meaningful way to the conversation. They might get lost in the middle of the conversation and have trouble getting back into the conversation. Your loved one might have difficulty with vocabulary, both in understanding others and in producing words themselves. You might hear your loved one talking in ways you do not understand, or they might repeat back the last few words or sounds you have made in ways that do not mean anything to you. They might call things by the incorrect names; for example, they might use incorrect pronouns or just describe an object when they cannot recall the correct name of the object: "You know, the little red, round, sweet things you make a pie out of," or they might call a watch a *wrist clock*. Other symptoms of language deficits are discussed in detail in chapter 5 about Aphasia.

Changes in Mood and Personality

Dementia can cause changes in mood and personality. Your loved one might become anxious, sad, lonely, frustrated, suspicious, depressed, hostile, or violent. They may have difficulty getting along or trusting people they have known for a long time. Home can be a place that is less emotionally challenging, although it can be a lonely place for your loved one.

Using Poor Judgment

Using poor judgment may become a problem for people who suffer from dementia. This can become evident when they become suspicious and accuse others of stealing from them when they misplace things or just become confused. They might also give valuable things away to strangers or charities and not remember doing this later. Poor judgment can also become evident in behaviors like eating inedible objects and playing with family pets in unsafe ways.

Social Withdrawal

Your loved one may begin to experience social withdraw and isolation. They may feel suspicious of others or become frightened from past experiences and home is where they feel safest. They may have difficulty remembering how to participate in their favorite hobbies or unable to understand their favorite sports anymore.

Inappropriate Behaviors

Behaviors may become inappropriate by way of being aggressive or hostile or even violent. Your loved one may not be able to tolerate frustration and may argue with you or strangers. Inappropriate sexual behaviors are common, as impulse-control becomes poor.

Inability to Learn or Remember New Information

Someone suffering from dementia might be unable to learn new information and might need to ask the same question many times and still might have difficulty making use of the information. You may need to continue to tell your loved one your name as you are visiting, or they may continue to ask you every few minutes where their deceased spouse is.

Paranoia and Hallucinations

Delusions, visual hallucinations, and audio hallucinations can occur with dementia. Some people suffering from dementia might think they need to "go home," or they may think a long lost loved one is in the room with them. They may see people who have died many years ago, or they may hear the voices of long-lost relatives. This can be a comforting experience for them, or it can be frightening.

Sun Downing

Sun downing is a phenomenon occurring with patients with dementia that causes their symptoms to increase when the sun begins to go down. You may notice your loved one will become more anxious or agitated during dusk, but their symptoms might begin to subside after dark. It is sometimes helpful to turn on extra lights during this time and engage your loved one in conversation to keep the focus on something other than the ambient environment.

Clinical Case Example of Bea

Bea is a seventy-six-year-old Caucasian woman who has lived with her husband in a suburban area most of her life. Bea's husband passed away six months ago, and since then she has been living in their large home alone. Bea's daughter lives nearby and has arranged for twenty-four-hour in-home care for Bea. Bea has exhibited difficulty with activities that require planning like shopping, preparing meals, housekeeping, and getting lost when she goes out of the house. Her behavior can be somewhat inappropriate; for example, she asks her caregivers explicit questions about their sex lives and tells waitresses they are overweight and not attractive. She has no language impairment and retains the ability to read and write. Bea has become more agitated and isolated recently with what appears to be a sudden onset of symptoms. What is more likely the case is that her husband was helping her to get through her day; therefore, her symptoms were less noticeable to others, but now that she doesn't have her husband to help her, her symptoms are more noticeable to others and probably to herself as well.

Bea exhibits severe disorientation when she first wakes up in the morning, and her caregivers spend about an hour orienting her to person, place, and time: she will ask a few questions about where she is and who she is and what time and date it is, over and over. After about an hour, she becomes oriented and just doesn't need to continue asking these questions. Bea is less confused during the daytime and is willing to go out to the market and around town with her caregivers; although she does get lost and confused, her experience is less frightening for her when she is with her caregivers. Bea's cognitive abilities and orientation begin to decline around evening, as it begins to get dark, and she starts to get more confused, agitated, and frightened. This is known as sun downing.

It is during this period that Bea can become completely disoriented, and she can become aggressive and violent. She sometimes goes into different rooms in her home and does not recognize her own things. She begins to take her things out of the drawers and cupboards and throw them away. This inability to recognize her own things and to remember owning them causes suspicion about her experience of herself and others, which in turn leads to agitation, aggression, and fear. When this cycle starts, her caregivers do not try to stop her, but rather they remove anything in her close environment that could be dangerous to her and just try to provide safety until the sun downing passes. There is risk of causing an already suspicious person to become more aggressive or violent with almost any intervention at this time.

For many patients, sun downing passes and its symptoms of increased anxiety, agitation, and aggression subside after the dusk passes and dark sets in. It is sometimes possible to expedite this process by keeping extra lights on before and during dusk and to give your loved one activities to do during this time to keep their mind occupied. If possible, spending time with your loved one in a room without windows during the evening hours might also help decrease symptoms of sun downing.

Middle Stage Symptoms (Moderate Dementia)

The amount of time someone stays in any stage of dementia depends partly on the type of dementia they have and other health factors; this is something a health-care provider can determine. Generally, people with dementia will spend more time in the beginning stages and less time in the final stages.

As your loved one moves on to the middle stage, their symptoms become more severe. For example, if they had difficulty with language, it will become more difficult for them to communicate. If they had difficulty with directions, they might begin to experience severe rather than mild confusion. It will become more difficult for them to keep their experience hidden, and you will begin to look back and understand that your loved one had been experiencing dementia all along.

It is important during this time to encourage your loved one to visit their medical doctor to receive a diagnosis and understand what is going on with their health. This is the time to complete legal documents to determine how they would like their medical decisions to be made should he become incapacitated.

Late-Stage Symptoms (Severe Dementia)

As your loved one progresses into late-stage dementia, their symptoms will become so severe they will not be able to take care of themselves, and you will need assistance taking care of them. You won't be able to have a conversation with them for more than a few minutes, and the content might not be meaningful. Dementia will completely take hold of their life in most areas of daily functioning.

Your loved one's short-term and long-term memory will become so impaired that they'll have difficulty recognizing family members, close friends, and neighbors whom they have known for a long time. They'll be completely dependent on others for daily needs like food preparation, toileting, bathing, and dressing. They will experience urinary and stool incontinence. Severe disorientation will become a problem, as will wandering off and getting lost. They'll experience severe behavior and personality changes including hostility, aggressiveness, and violence. Communication will become impaired to the extent that it may become impossible to understand them. Finally, difficulty swallowing may cause choking and difficulty eating, while mechanical feeding may be necessary.

Clinical Case Example of Anne

Anne is an eighty-two-year-old Caucasian woman who lives with her daughter and son-in-law in their suburban home in North America. Anne is in excellent physical health, with the exception of successful recent cataract surgery in her left eye. Anne had lived independently since the death of her husband thirty-two years ago. Now, at age eighty-two, she has moved in with her daughter and son-in-law at their request due to her significant confusion, global aphasia, disorientation at night, and difficulty remembering things: for example, forgetting to turn off the stove (thereby causing a minor kitchen fire) and, on several occasions, her needing the assistance of neighbors because she forgot how to get home from the store.

Upon entering Anne's home, it is clear she is quite gracious and warm. Conversation with her begins as it would with most other people, and one would be pressed to know she is suffering from moderate dementia. However, as the details of the conversation with her become more in-depth and complicated, Anne is unable to remember what has been said and becomes "lost" and unable to contribute meaningfully to the conversation. Additionally, Anne has no insight into her impairment; therefore, she can become frustrated with her conversation partner and, at times, somewhat aggressive.

Anne uses neologisms (made-up words) and at times, due to her receptive and productive aphasia, she will describe the words she is looking for. Again, she suffers from impaired insight, and when her listener fails to understand what she is trying to communicate, she can become frustrated and aggressive, even hostile because she fails to understand why her conversation partner will not continue to carry on the conversation with her.

Due in part to this process, at times Anne experiences paranoia. As a consequence of her language impairment, her failure to be understood, her impaired insight, and the way in which she attempts to make sense of all this, she sometimes believes others around her have orchestrated all these elements because they are trying to harm her. At these times, Anne can become frightened and hostile and even violent in an attempt to protect herself.

Anne's daughter reports that some mornings, she finds that Anne has visited the kitchen and opened drawers and cupboards and removed items, some food items and some nonfood items, and emptied the contents into plates and bowls. She reports that it appears that Anne has tried to eat these items. Furthermore, when Anne awakes in the morning, not only does she have no recollection of her behavior during the night, but also she becomes defensively hostile about being questioned and accused.

Sometimes during the early evening, Anne can be found walking from room to room, calling out her deceased husband's name as though she is looking for him. Her daughter reports that when she attempts to help her or to explain that her father has died, it has no apparent effect on her mother, and she continues "looking" for her deceased husband: just walking from room to room, calling out to him.

Sometimes at night, Anne gets out of her bed and wanders about the house crying because she is confused and cannot figure out if it is daytime or nighttime. Her circadian rhythm and sleep architecture are unstable, and she cannot sleep through most nights. She usually goes into her daughter's bedroom and gets into bed with her and sleeps there for several hours until the next time she wakes. The next time she wakes, when she sees her daughter and son-in-law sleeping and she feels safe, she usually goes back into her own bedroom and continues sleeping.

Anne can be difficult to soothe because of her impaired insight. She responds positively to being treated like an adored child and the use of endearing names like "princess" and "sunshine." Although her daughter reports this can sometimes be difficult for her (to call her own mother by the very pet names Anne once used to soothe her), when she does it is comforting when nothing else can soothe her. She also responds positively to being touched on her arm and holding hands and someone stroking her hair: generally just being "adored" as you would a favorite child.

3. Doctors and Treatments

The umbrella term of *health care professional* encompasses virtually anyone who provides either medical or mental health care to someone who seeks this type of care. Usually, a professional's education is reflected in their title, but this can often be misleading. Additionally, what health-care professionals believe their respective areas of expertise are can often be a point of disagreement among other health-care professionals.

So, who is best qualified to diagnose and take care of your loved one? Often there will be many people providing "team" care for your loved one. But there are going to be several people who are vital to your team. You will need a geriatric physician, a geriatric psychiatrist, a neuropsychologist, and a clinical geropsychologist or clinical psychologist.

A physician who specializes in geriatrics is one who will be able to treat the physical components of your loved one's dementia and related disorders. For example, with vascular dementia, associated risk factors for stroke need to be treated and managed as well as pain. A geriatric psychiatrist will be able to treat your loved one's psychiatric symptoms of dementia: for example, agitation, mood changes, and hallucinations. A neuropsychologist will be able to perform a battery of neuropsych assessments to determine the location and extent of the damage and type of dementia as well as provide a prognosis for your loved one. The clinical geropsychologist and clinical psychologist will be able to determine day-to-day functional impairment as well as individual strengths your loved one can use to maintain the highest possible quality of life for as long as possible. The clinical geropsychologist and clinical psychologist, by assessing most effective living placements, behavioral interventions, and treatment modalities, can also be helpful with developing individual treatment plans that will help your loved one maintain as much independence as possible.

These are the vital members of your treatment team, and the additional care providers should be individualized depending on your loved one's needs and where they are in the progression of their illness. It can be confusing to determine exactly who each health-care provider is and how to identify them because there are so many to sort through. Therefore, I have provided detailed descriptions of how to recognize a geriatric physician, geriatric psychiatrist, neuropsychologist, clinical geropsychologist, and a clinical psychologist.

Geriatric Physician

Internal or family medicine is a specialty of medicine while geriatrics is a subspecialty of both internal and family medicine. This subspecialty requires additional education and training and certification in most states. Geriatric medicine is the delivery of medical care to the elderly population with a focus on prevention and treatment of disease and disabilities in the elderly. Subspecialties within geriatric medicine include:

- cardiogeriatrics (heart disease)
- geriatric nephrology (kidney disease)
- geriatric dentistry (dental disorders)
- geriatric rehabilitation (physical therapy)
- geriatric oncology (cancerous tumor)
- geriatric rheumatology (joints and soft tissue disorders)

- geriatric neurology (neurologic disorders)
- geriatric dermatology (skin disorders)
- geriatric emergency medicine
- geriatric pharmacotherapy
- geriatric intensive-care unit: (a special type of intensive care unit dedicated to critically ill elderly)
- geriatric nursing (nursing of elderly patients).
- geriatric nutrition
- geriatric pain management

As people age, their physical needs become different, and this is what sets geriatric medicine apart from adult medicine. For example, wear and tear on the body is a more prevalent issue in geriatric medicine as with smokers or patients who have neglected issues like diet and exercise. Additionally, as we age our organ systems begin to decline. For example, renal impairment might be a normal symptom of aging; however, renal failure is not. Geriatric medicine distinguishes between normal aging processes and medical illnesses.

Partly due to normal decline, the elderly become more at risk for complications from mild issues to become severe issues. For example, a slight fever in an elderly adult might cause confusion or disorientation, which might in turn contribute to a fall that may result in a bone fracture.

Finally, geriatric physicians are trained for the special needs of the elderly regarding medications. Medications are metabolized through the kidney or liver, which may be compromised in the elderly and cause a slower excretion process of medications. This may cause medications to stay in their systems longer, which produces the potential for drug overdose. Additionally, the elderly often take more than one medication, often prescribed by more than one doctor. Combine this with a possible over-the-counter regimen, and many elderly patients have the potential for medication interactions and overdose.

Geriatric physicians are trained to recognize impairments with quality-of-life issues like the patient's ability to bathe themselves, feed themselves, dress themselves, mobility issues, and communication issues. The geriatric physician can therefore consider these important factors when making a recommendation about your loved one's care: for example, when weighing the risk and benefit of invasive medical procedures like surgery and post-op care and recovery.

Geriatric Psychiatrist

A psychiatrist is a doctor who has been to medical school for four years and has then specialized in psychiatry. Geriatric psychiatry is a subspecialty of psychiatry, and in many states, board certification with the American Board of Psychiatry and Neurology is required. Geriatric psychiatry is concerned with prevention and treatment of mental disorders of the elderly population, of which dementia and depression are two common issues.

Elderly patients don't usually have one mental health diagnosis; more often it is comorbid (occurring alongside) with several diagnoses, some regarding mental health and some physical health. Therefore, a more comprehensive diagnostic approach, one which encompasses their psychological and physical needs, is effective with this population.

Because the geriatric psychiatrist went to medical school, he is in a special position on the health-care team. He has expertise from both a medical perspective and a psychological perspective and can communicate information to other members of the team and make recommendations to primary-care doctors when mental illness is involved in the treatment. The geriatric psychiatrist can also supervise other members of the treatment team when your loved one moves into a facility or needs a higher level of care at home.

Neuropsychologist

A neuropsychologist is a psychologist who has received special training before and after licensure regarding cortical structures and their functions and how they impact psychological issues and behavior. Neuropsychologists are trained in neurological assessment, which are batteries of tests that help the neuropsychologist determine structural and functional damage to the brain as a result of injury or illness.

The neurophychologist will implement a battery of assessments that are designed to evaluate one cognitive process correlated to the performance on the test. Examples of standardized tests neurospychologists might use are the Wechsler Adult Intelligence Scale, Wechsler Intelligence Scale for Children, Halstead-Reitan Neuropsychological Battery, Wisconsin Card Sorting Test, Controlled Oral Word Association, Minnesota Multiphasic Personality Inventory, and the Extended Mental Status Examination.

Standardized assessments require the patient to have the ability to read, write, and understand language, which is sometimes not a possibility for all patients. Therefore, neuropsychologists also use neuroimaging for assessment. These include Functional Magnetic Resonance Imaging (FMRI) and Computerized Axial Tomography scan (CAT scan) and Positron Emission Tomography scan (PET scan). Additionally, neurophychologists regularly make use of equipment measuring the magnetic activity within the brain produced by the nervous system. This may include electro-encephalography (EEG) or magneto-encephalography (MEG).

Clinical Geropsychologist and Clinical Psychologist

A clinical psychologist has graduated from a doctoral-degree-granting graduate program of clinical psychology, conducted original research—a dissertation—and has completed two full-time years of supervised clinical work before being able to sit for licensure examinations. Geropsychology is a subspecialty of clinical psychology, and in most states, additional training and board certification are required.

Geropsychology has a focus on the concerns of the elderly population and the final developmental issues of life. These concerns might include maintaining independence and achieving the highest level of happiness and highest quality of life possible for the longest amount of time possible.

Geropsychologists and clinical psychologists administer and interpret psychological and diagnostic assessment, psychotherapy, treatment planning, research, and consultation, provide expert testimony, and teach. Geropsychologists work primarily with the elderly, while a clinical psychologist may work with the elderly as well as with adults, adolescents, children, families, and couples.

Clinical psychologists are trained in the administration and interpretation of psychological assessments from which they are able to make diagnostic impressions. Some of the more common psychological assessments they use are intelligence tests, personality tests, neuropsychological tests, and clinical interview.

There are several ways to locate the specific types of doctor you are looking for. For example, you can contact local hospitals or contact your insurance carrier for a list of their covered providers. You can also do a Google search on the internet and follow-up any doctor you are interested in by contacting their licensing board to look for any restrictions on their license. You can also contact your state licensing board for lists of licensed doctors in your state. Physicians and psychiatrists are licensed by the same regulatory board and separate from psychologists who are licensed with the same regulatory board in most states.

You might also talk to friends and family members who have had experiences with their doctors- either good or bad experiences are all good information. Contact your family doctor for a recommendation for a specialist.

Treatments for Dementia

FDA-Approved Medications

Acetylcholinesterase inhibitors

"Donepezil (Aricept), Rivastigmine (Exelon) and Galantamine Hydrobromide (Razadyne) and Rivastigmine (Exelon) : these drugs are approved by the United States Food and Drug Association (FDA) for the treatment of dementia induced by Alzheimer's disease. They work by boosting levels of a chemical messenger involved in memory and judgment. Side effects can include nausea, vomiting, and diarrhea. Although primarily used as Alzheimer's drugs, they're also used to treat vascular, Parkinson's, and Lewy body dementias" (Mayo Clinic).

Memantine (Namenda)

"This drug for Alzheimer's disease works by regulating the activity of glutamate, another chemical messenger involved in all brain function, including learning and memory. Its most common side effect is dizziness. Some research has shown that combining Memantine with a cholinesterase inhibitor may have even better results. Although primarily used to treat Alzheimer's disease, it may help improve symptoms in other dementias" (Mayo Clinic).

Off-Label Prescriptions

Antidepressant drugs

Because depression can begin with the onset of dementia or become worse with the symptoms of dementia and because depression can generally impair cognitive and behavioral function, treatment with antidepressant drugs is therefore indicated. Depression symptoms can sometimes be effectively managed in patients with dementia.

Antipsychotic drugs

Psychotic symptoms can be effectively managed with both typical and atypical antipsychotic medications. The use of any antipsychotic medication can increase the risk of death in dementia-related psychosis, and the use of antipsychotic medication is therefore considered off-label use.

Anxiolytic drugs

Using medications like benzodiazepines to treat anxiety symptoms in patients with dementia is often avoided because these drugs can increase agitation and are likely to worsen cognitive problems and may increase agitation.

Other medications

Although no standard treatment for dementia exists, some symptoms can be effectively managed. Additional treatments aim to reduce the risk factors for further brain damage.

Your prescriber may use different medications to address the progress of underlying causes of dementia-related symptoms. For example, medications might be used to treat high blood pressure to prevent a stroke, which will reduce further symptoms of increased dementia. With patients who have dementia, medication might also be used to manage symptoms like insomnia and behavioral problems; other medications might also address pain management for people with dementia.

Alternative Medicine

When you are considering using alternative remedies to treat any medical or psychological condition, you should proceed with caution. Not only are you using something that has not been tested through clinical trials, but you are also using valuable time, possibly without efficacious treatment. Dietary supplements, vitamins, and herbal remedies are not sold under a standard measurement; therefore, it is difficult to know exactly how much you are taking each time. Alternative medications might also interact with prescription medications, so always consult with your prescriber before taking anything in conjunction with what you have been prescribed.

Some of the more popular alternatives for Alzheimer's disease and other forms of dementia are described below.

Vitamin E

"Some studies have shown that vitamin E can slow the progression of Alzheimer's disease, while other studies have shown no benefit. Some doctors warn against taking large doses of vitamin E, especially if you're taking blood thinners, because of an increased risk of bleeding" (Mayo Clinic, 2010).

Omega-3 fatty acids

Omega-3 fatty acids have been associated with health benefits, including decreased heart disease, reduced risk of stroke, and lower risk of developing dementia. The FDA recommendations regarding omega-3s are not to exceed a combined total of 3 grams of DHA or EPA a day. Omega-3s are theorized to increase the vascular health; thus, reducing the risk of certain vascular dementias. It is also possible that omega-3s play a role in preventing symptoms of depression (Mayo Clinic, 2010).

Coenzyme Q10

A naturally occurring antioxidant that is essential for normal body function, coenzyme Q10 has had little research of its benefits for treating dementia. Idebenone, a synthetic compound resembling coenzyme Q10, was tested for Alzheimer's disease but didn't show favorable results. There is little known about safe dosage; however, reports about overdosing have been recorded, with effects including bruising, bleeding, and lowering of blood glucose (Mayo Clinic, 2010).

Ginkgo

Ginkgo biloba has been reported to have been used for its antioxidant and anti-inflammatory benefit; however, clinical studies have yet to confirm the efficacy of these beliefs, and there might be dangers of interactions with other medications (Mayo Clinic, 2010).

Huperzine A

Made from naturally occurring vegetation, Huperzine A seems to work in ways similar to cholinesterase inhibitors. Therefore, increased risk of possible harmful side effects exists when taking prescription medications, which should not be taken together with Huperzine A (Mayo Clinic, 2010).

4. Putting Legal Affairs in Order

Once your loved one receives a diagnosis of dementia, one of the first things you should do is to put their legal affairs in order. Waiting too long to do this can be risky because dementia is a progressive disease with increasing cognitive impairment, and waiting too long can be problematic when legal affairs are concerned.

If your loved one has already made legal arrangements concerning their wishes about their health care in the event they become unable to make these decisions for himself, perhaps you should review their decisions to be sure they are not outdated. Talk with your loved one to be sure you understand their wishes before their cognitive decline becomes too severe to make these decisions for himself.

Even if your loved one has made decisions about their end-of-life choices, they might not have made a will, created a living trust, or written an advanced health-care directive. Now is the time to put their wishes in writing.

There are several documents your loved one will need, and these will vary from state to state. Generally, you will need to prepare health-care documents that communicate your loved one's wishes should they become unable to communicate for themselves, and you will need to prepare financial documents that communicate your loved one's wishes around financial management.

Advanced Health Care Directive

One necessary health-care document that is required in almost every state is the advanced health-care directive. This document explains the wishes of a person regarding his health care and is executed once he becomes unable to communicate for himself. Advance directives for health care include living wills, the durable power of attorney for health care, and do not resuscitate (DNR) orders.

A living will documents the person's wishes about specific medical circumstances that may require medical treatment or life-sustaining procedures and treatment. This document provides the framework for end-of-life care and for a patient's wish to die with dignity. This document can also protect the physician and facility from recourse for withholding life-sustaining procedures or for withdrawing life supportive treatment.

Durable Power of Attorney

A durable power of attorney for health care is a document used for communicating wishes regarding future health-care decisions; in addition to health-care decisions, this document also is used to designate the specific person to carry out those wishes and make decisions should the medical situation become unclear and if the patient is unable to make decisions for himself. This document is different from a normal power of attorney, which would become invalid when the person becomes mentally incapacitated. The durable power of attorney is for the specific situation of when a person becomes incapacitated because of mental defect. It can be very complicated with specific details about what the agent can and cannot do with specific time limits and limiting circumstances regarding his power of action. The agent might have the final decision regarding many health-care options; for example, he might be given power to decide if and when discharge of health-care providers will occur, or when removing the patient from an institution will occur; he may choose to refuse or agree to various treatments; he may have access to medical records; or he may make decisions about making anatomical gifts.

Because of the rigorous demands on the designated agent, the person serving in this position should not only be someone who knows the person well but also someone who can do well under extreme pressure. In most states, the agent will make decisions regarding end-of-life care—like where the patient will end their life—unless this is specifically spelled out in the advanced health care directive. The agent will be able to make decisions about where care will be provided—in a hospice facility, a hospital, or at home—and if life-supportive efforts will be made or continued or discontinued, like the use of a feeding tube.

Because these types of decisions can be so difficult and have such overwhelming consequences for the patient and family members, it is recommended that an alternate agent be designated as well, in case the primary agent finds himself having a hard time or needing assistance with some of these decisions, or is unavailable to make some of these decisions.

Do not Resuscitate Order

The do not resuscitate (DNR) order is a document in which specific instructions are given to health-care providers to not perform emergency measures to extend or save the life of the patient in medical situations where the patient's life could be saved or prolonged if these procedures were used.

Financial Documents

There are several types of documents to communicate the wishes of the person regarding financial management and estate planning that should be completed before he becomes unable to communicate for himself. Some of these documents include the durable power of attorney for finances, wills, and living trusts. As is the case with the health-care documents, these financial documents must also be prepared before the person becomes mentally incapacitated by his illness.

The durable power of attorney is a document that provides an agent the power to make decisions regarding financial affairs on behalf of the afflicted person. This document is expected to be executed in the future, when the person becomes incapacitated by their illness, and the document is still in effect after the person becomes mentally incapacitated (unlike some other legal documents).

The will is a document that designates specifically how the person's assets will be divided up among the beneficiaries after the person's death. For example, you may find things like who will care for minor children, trusts for estates, where specific gifts will be donated, and burial and funeral plans.

The living trust is a document in which a "grantor" creates a trust and designates a person to serve as trustee and follow the trust's terms after the grantor dies. This is where the assets are managed for the beneficiary of the trust. This arrangement is created while the grantor is still alive rather than at his death. The main advantages of a living trust are that not only can it include most types of property, but it can also provide instructions for its disposition after the grantor's death. The trustee can also be named as the health-care agent through a durable power of attorney for health care.

Planning for final arrangements with your loved one might also be something to consider. This can help reduce a sense of anxiety for family members and for the person who is ill. This is a conversation that might be important to many people because for some, the way in which burial takes place is very important and if this is not attended to properly, then the person will feel they cannot pass on the way they need to.

Your loved one may need time to think about all of these plans, and in time they might want to revisit their decisions for a sense of closure. This is a good idea. Encourage your loved one to have additional conversations with their doctor, their legal representation, and their family members for as long as their mental health permits.

Your Loved one's Household Budget

There will come a time in your loved one's care when you will need to arrange to take care of their budget for the daily living expenses. This will encompass things like paying their bills, managing bank accounts, managing health insurance and healthcare providers, and managing any other daily or monthly needs and expenses they incur. This task can be very different for each person, and you might be surprised when you discover what this entails for your loved one. Sit down together and figure out what needs to be attended to, just like your own budget. This might be a work in progress for a while, probably just like your own budget can be sometimes. But this is possible, and you will get through this too.

These documents are complicated and are best done with the expert advice of legal counsel. However, many of these documents can be completed through the assistance of interactive online Web sites like www.legalzoom.com and are also available as blank forms that may be purchased or downloaded free from online Web sites like www.lawdepot.com.

Once the pressing matter of these crucial legal concerns has been addressed, you will better **be** able to return your focus to understanding your loved one's dementia and how best to help her.

Examples of Legal Documents

The following examples have been reprinted with permission of the copyright owner and are intended to serve only as examples to the reader. "These documents are examples only of the estate planning documents that you may require to plan for potential incapacity during your lifetime. State law varies and therefore your state may require different language in your planning documents than the language provided here. You should always consult an attorney licensed to practice law in your state to make certain your documents are compliant with the law where you reside (McCurdy, 2011)."

Example: **DURABLE POWER OF ATTORNEY FOR PROPERTY FOR JANE DOE**

KNOW ALL MEN BY THESE PRESENTS, that I, JANE DOE, currently a resident of _____ hereby appoint, AGENT (My agent, who currently resides at), to serve, as my true and lawful attorney-in-fact (sometimes referred to as "my agent") to act in, manage, and conduct all of my affairs and for that purpose, in my name and on my behalf, to do and execute any or all of the following acts, deeds, and matters to be effective, only if I become incapacitated as determined by two (2) physicians.

This Durable Power of Attorney for Property shall not be terminated by my mental or physical incompetence.

I intend by this power of attorney to eliminate the need for a court-supervised guardianship or conservatorship. Should my intent be defeated, I ask that my agent or such person as my agent may nominate be appointed as guardian or conservator of my estate and be excused from bond. I further intend that this Durable Power of Attorney for Property be exercisable in any state or jurisdiction in which I may have any property or interest in property.

1.   To ask, demand, sue for, recover, and receive all sums of money, debts, dues, goods, wares, merchandise, chattels, effects, and things of whatsoever nature or description that now are or hereafter shall be or become due, owing, payable, or belonging to me, and upon receipt thereof, or of any part thereof, to make, sign, execute, and deliver such receipts, releases, or other discharges for the same as my agent shall deem advisable.

2.   To settle and/or to pay or receive any account whatsoever wherein I now am or at any time hereafter may be in any way interested or concerned.

3.   To receive every sum of money that now is or hereafter shall be due or belonging to me by virtue of any mortgage, deed to secure debt, or other security instrument, and on receipt of the full amount secured thereby, to execute a good and sufficient release or other discharge thereof.

4.   To compromise or make allowances to any person for or with respect to any debt whatsoever that now is or at any time hereafter shall become due and payable by me, and to take and receive any composition or dividend thereof, and to give releases or other discharges for the whole or any part of such debts or demands, or to settle, compromise, or submit to arbitration every such debt or demand and every other right, matter, and thing due by, to, or concerning me, as my agent shall deem appropriate, and for that purpose, to enter into, execute, and deliver such releases, compromises, or other instruments as my agent may deem advisable.

5. To commence, prosecute, discontinue, or defend all actions or other legal proceedings involving any matter in which I may have an interest.

6. To enter into and upon all real estate of mine and to manage and improve the same, or any part thereof, and to repair or otherwise improve or alter and insure any buildings thereon.

7. To contract with any person for leasing all or any real estate for such periods, at such rents and subject to such conditions as my agent shall deem advisable, to let any such person into possession thereof, to execute all such leases and contracts as shall be necessary or proper, to give notice of eviction to any tenant or occupant thereof, to receive and recover from all or any number of the tenants and occupants thereof all rents and sums of money that now are or hereafter shall become due and payable in respect thereof, and on nonpayment of any part or all thereof, to take all necessary or proper means and proceedings for terminating the tenancy or occupancy of such tenants or occupants and for evicting the tenants or occupants and recovering the possession thereof.

8. To sell, either at public or private sale, or exchange any part or parts of my real or personal property for such consideration and upon such terms and conditions as my agent shall deem advisable, to execute and deliver good and sufficient deeds or other instruments for the conveyance or transfer of the same, with such covenants of warranty or otherwise as my agent shall deem appropriate, and to give good and effectual receipts for all or part of the purchase price or other consideration. The power to sell shall include the power to dispose of United States Treasury securities, including, but not limited to, United States Treasury bonds and notes.

9. To dispose of any of my property if in the discretion of my agent it shall require greater resources to retain the asset than to dispose of it.

10. To deposit any money that may come into the possession of my agent while acting in such capacity with any bank or banker, either in my name or that of my agent, and to withdraw any of such money or any other money to which I am or I or my agent hereafter shall be entitled, and to employ said money as my agent shall deem advisable in the payment of any debts, obligations, interest, taxes, assessments, insurance, and any expenses due and payable or to become due and payable by or on my account or otherwise for my use and benefit.

11. To purchase or invest in, either in my name or in that of my agent, any stocks, shares, bonds, securities, or other property, real or personal, as my agent may deem proper, for cash or upon such terms as my agent may deem appropriate, and to receive and give receipts for any income or dividend arising from such investments.

12. To borrow for investments, purchases, or otherwise any sum or sums of money on such terms and with such security, whether real or personal property, as my agent may deem appropriate and for that purpose to execute all promissory notes, endorsements, guarantees, bonds, mortgages, security deeds, and other instruments that may be necessary or proper; and to enter into and execute in my name any guarantees, endorsements, suretyships, or other accommodations in regard to any partnership, venture, or corporation in which I may have an interest or otherwise as my agent may deem appropriate.

13. To engage, employ, and dismiss any agents, attorneys, accountants, clerks, servants, or other persons as my agent shall

deem appropriate to assist my agent in the performance of the powers granted herein, and to pay reasonable compensation for such services.

14. To vote at the meetings of stockholders or other meetings of any corporation, partnership, venture, or company or otherwise to act as my attorney or proxy or to execute any proxies or other instruments in respect of any stocks, bonds, securities, or other instruments now or hereafter held by me.

15. To enter into and sign, seal, execute, acknowledge, and deliver any contracts, options, deeds, or other instruments whatsoever, and to draw, accept, make, endorse, discount, or otherwise deal with any bills of exchange, checks, promissory notes, or other commercial or mercantile instruments for any or all of the purposes of this Durable Power of Attorney for Property.

16. To prepare, execute, and file federal, state, county, and municipal income, gift, property, estate, and other tax returns for me; to have full power to perform any and all acts that I could perform pertaining to tax matters, including, but not limited to, the power to receive and endorse checks in payment of any refund of taxes, penalties, or interest, to execute waivers of restrictions on assessment or collection of deficiencies in tax, to execute consents extending the statutory period for assessment or collection of taxes, to execute a closing agreement (under Internal Revenue Code ("I.R.C.") Section 7121), in respect of any tax liability or specific matter, to execute a protest to a determination of taxes, and to delegate authority or to substitute another agent.

17. My agent is authorized expressly and shall have the power to make nontaxable gifts and/or nontaxable transfers of any of my assets to any person, including gifts or transfers to or for the benefit of my agent hereunder. The term(s) "nontaxable

gifts" and/or "nontaxable transfers" shall be deemed to include the following types of transfers: (a) transfers that qualify for the marital deduction under I.R.C. Section 2523; (b) transfers that qualify for a charitable contribution deduction under I.R.C. Section 2522; and (c) transfers that are not subject to gift tax pursuant to the provisions of I.R.C. Sections 2503(b), (c), and (e). In addition and not in limitation of the preceding provisions of this paragraph 16, my agent is authorized expressly and shall have the power to make taxable gifts outright or in trust or otherwise to my children and/or their descendants. Notwithstanding the foregoing provisions of this paragraph, the total of all gifts and transfers to or for the benefit of any agent or co agent in any calendar year shall not exceed an amount equal to five percent (5%) of my net worth as of January 1 of the calendar year of the gift in question.

18. To act as my deputy or legal representative in obtaining access to, and to control the contents of, any safe, safety deposit box, or functional equivalent for which I have a right to access.

19. To renounce or disclaim, in whole or in part, any interest in property transferred or to be transferred to me or to which I have succeeded or may succeed by contract or operation of law, including the power to disclaim any power or other rights that I may have with respect to such property, regardless of whether such renunciation or disclaimer qualifies as a qualified disclaimer under federal or local law.

20. To prepare, execute, file and prosecute any claim I may have for benefits provided by the United States or any state or by any agency or subdivisions thereof; to provide such information or authorize the disclosure of such information respecting me and others as may be required in support thereof; to appear on

my behalf; and to take such further actions, appeals, complaints or other proceedings of any nature or kind whatsoever as may be necessary or appropriate to prosecute any claim for benefits, and to receive said benefits in my name or in the name of the agent as representative payee or otherwise, and to take all such other actions relating to any government benefits as I myself could do.

21. In general, to do all other acts, deeds, matters, and things whatsoever in or about my property and affairs, including waiving any right I may have or to concur with persons jointly interested with myself therein in doing all acts, deeds, matters, and things herein, either particularly or generally described, as fully and effectually to all intents and purposes as I could do in my own proper person if personally present.

If AGENT, my agent herein named, shall become unable or unwilling to serve as my agent hereunder, I appoint the following, each to act one at a time and in the order stated, to serve as my successor agent hereunder, and each such successor agent shall have all the same powers and authorities herein granted to the original agent appointed above:

a. SUCCESSOR AGENT (My agent, who currently resides at); and then,

b. SUCCESSOR AGENT (My agent, who currently resides at).

An individual shall be deemed to be unable or unwilling to serve or continue serving as an agent hereunder if: (1) such individual dies, is adjudicated incompetent by a court of competent jurisdiction, or notifies me, the agent(s) serving hereunder, and any successor agent(s) named herein in writing of such individual's inability or unwillingness to serve or continue serving as an agent hereunder; (2) two licensed medical doctors who are familiar with the physical and mental condition of such individual determine in a written instrument, a copy of which shall be delivered to me, to the agent(s) serving hereunder, and to such individual's successor agent(s) named herein, if any, that such individual at the time in question is unable or unwilling to serve or to continue serving as such agent; or (3) a court having the requisite jurisdiction determines for any reason that such individual is unable or unwilling to serve or to continue serving as such agent.

All successor agents hereunder shall have all the same powers and authorities herein granted to the original agent appointed above.

This power of attorney creates rights only. It does not create any obligation upon my agent to act. My agent shall not incur any liability to me or to anyone claiming through me for acting or refraining from acting under this power of attorney for any action or omission taken in good faith pursuant to this Durable Power of Attorney for Property; nor shall my agent be responsible for the actions of any other agent who may have earlier served as my agent.

All references in this Durable Power of Attorney for Property to section(s) of the Internal Revenue Code are to section(s) of the Internal Revenue Code of 1986 presently in force or as such section(s) and/or code from time to time hereafter may be amended or superseded.

IN WITNESS WHEREOF, I have hereunto set my hand and affixed my seal, this _____ day of _____, 20.

_____ (SEAL)

JANE DOE

Witnesses:

JANE DOE, the principal, has had an opportunity to read the above Durable Power of Attorney for Health Care and has signed said document in our presence. We, the undersigned, each being over eighteen (18) years of age, hereby witness the principal's signature at the request and in the presence of the principal, and in the presence of each other, the day and year above set out. We further declare that we are not related to the principal by blood, marriage or adoption, and, to the best of my knowledge, we are not entitled to any part of the estate of the principal under a currently existing will or by operation of law, we are not the attending physician of the principal or an employee of a health care facility in which the principal is a patient, nor do we have a claim against the principal or the principal's estate now or after the principal's death.

Witnesses: Addresses:

_____ (Signature) _____

_____ (Print Name) _____

_____ (Signature) _____

_____ (Print Name) _____

STATE OF   §§
COUNTY OF   §

BEFORE ME, the undersigned authority, person-
ally appeared JANE DOE to me well known or producing
_____ as identification, being by
me first duly sworn, who deposes and says that she executed the
above and foregoing Durable Power of Attorney for Property for
the uses and purposes therein expressed.

WITNESS my hand and seal at the City of _____ ,
County of _____ , State of, on this day of _____ , 20.

Notary Public

My Commission Expires:

YOU MAY, BUT ARE NOT REQUIRED TO, REQUEST
YOUR AGENT AND SUCCESSOR AGENTS TO PROVIDE
SPECIMEN SIGNATURES BELOW. IF YOU INCLUDE
SPECIMEN SIGNATURES IN THIS POWER OF ATTORNEY,
YOU MUST COMPLETE THE CERTIFICATION OPPOSITE
THE SIGNATURES OF THE AGENTS.

Example : **DURABLE POWER OF ATTORNEY FOR
HEALTH CARE FOR JANE DOE**

(also known as, Advanced Health Care Directive in Some
States)

DURABLE POWER OF ATTORNEY FOR HEALTH CARE
made this _____ day of _____ , 20.

When a Loved One at Home has Dementia:

1. I, JANE DOE, currently a resident of
, hereby appoint, AGENT (My agent, who currently resides at
_____), as my attorney-in-fact (my "agent") to act for and in my name, place, and stead, and on my behalf, for the specific purposes hereinafter described, only if I become incapacitated as determined by two (2) physicians.

   a. To act for me and in my name, in any way I could act in person, to make any and all decisions for me concerning my personal care, medical treatment, hospitalization, and health care, and to require, withhold, or withdraw any type of medical treatment or procedure, even though my death may ensue.

   b. My agent shall have the same access to my medical records that I have, including the right to disclose the contents to others.

   c. My agent also shall have full power to make a disposition of any part or all of my body for medical purposes, authorize an autopsy of my body, and direct the disposition of my remains; provided, however, my agent shall not be authorized to make any disposition of my body and/or my remains that is inconsistent with any direction that I may make in my Last Will and Testament, Disposition of Remains or in a memorandum, wholly in my own handwriting left at my death, signed by me and dated after the date of this Durable Power of Attorney for Healthcare listing specific instructions as to the disposition of my body and/or my remains.

   d. As to all matters herein described or contemplated, to give oral or written consent to the performance of any one or all of such medical applications to be made.

e. To agree to and to hold, in my name, any doctor, techni-
cian, hospital, or other medical personage free and harmless from
any claim, demand, or suit for damages from any injury or com-
plication that may result from such treatment or medical applica-
tion to me.

f. To do and perform all and every act that I legally may
do through an agent concerning the subject matter of this power
of attorney, and every proper power necessary to carry out the
purposes for which this Durable Power of Attorney for Health
Care is granted, with full power of substitution and revocation. I
hereby ratify and affirm that which my agent lawfully shall do or
cause to be done by virtue of the powers herein conferred upon
my agent.

2. The powers granted above shall not include the following
powers or shall be subject to the following rules or limitations:
　　No Limitation　　　Initialed

3. The powers granted above shall not include the following
powers or shall be subject to the following rules or limitations:

a. I do not want my life to be prolonged nor do I want life-
sustaining or death-delaying treatment to be provided or continued if my agent believes the burdens of the treatment outweigh
the expected benefits. I want my agent to consider the relief of
suffering, the expense involved, and the quality as well as the possible extension of my life in making decisions concerning life-sustaining or death-delaying treatment. Except as provided above in
paragraph 2, I expressly authorize my agent to obtain or terminate

any type of health care, including the withdrawal of nourishment and fluids and other life-sustaining or death-delaying measures.
Initialed

b. I want my life to be prolonged and I want life-sustaining or death-delaying treatment to be provided or continued unless I am in a coma, including a persistent vegetative state, which my attending physician believes to be irreversible, in accordance with reasonable medical standards at the time of reference. If and when I have suffered such an irreversible coma, I want life-sustaining or death-delaying treatment to be withheld or discontinued.
Initialed

c. I want my life to be prolonged to the greatest extent possible without regard to my condition, the chances I have for recovery, or the cost of the procedures.
Initialed

4. This power of attorney shall become effective immediately upon a determination of my incapacity by two (2) physicians, one of which has examined me within one day preceding certification of such and the other of which must be a neurologist, neurosurgeon or other physician with expertise in cognitive functioning as provided by the Annotated Code of STATE .

5. If AGENT, the agent hereinabove named, shall become unable or unwilling to serve as my agent hereunder, I name the following, each to act one at a time and in the order stated, to serve as my successor agent under this document:

a. SUCCESSOR AGENT (My Son, who currently resides at_____); and then,

b. SUCCESSOR AGENT (My Daughter, who currently resides at _____).

6. All successor agent(s) shall have all the same powers and authorities as are granted to the original agent(s) hereunder. If at any time more than two individuals shall serve together as my agent hereunder, (1) all decisions to be made hereunder shall be made by the majority vote of such individuals, and (2) any writing signed by a majority of my agents hereunder shall be as valid and effective for all purposes as if signed by all such agents.

7. If a guardian of my person is to be appointed, I nominate AGENT to serve as such guardian, and if AGENT shall be unable or unwilling to serve or to continue as my guardian, I nominate the following persons, each to act one at a time and in the order stated, to serve as such guardian:

a. SUCCESSOR AGENT (My   agent, who currently resides at_____); and then,

b. SUCCESSOR AGENT (My   agent, who currently resides at_____).

8. I also have executed a Living Will. I understand that by statute this Durable Power of Attorney for Health Care supersedes the Living Will as long as there is an agent able and/or willing to act under this power. My directions concerning my health

care and the withdrawal of life-sustaining or death-delaying treatment set forth in my Living Will, by statute, may be more limited than the powers I am granting to my agent under this Durable Power of Attorney for Health Care. I do not want the more limited directions set forth in my Living Will to restrict the decisions my agent may make pursuant to this Durable Power of Attorney for Health Care, but, rather, I want my agent to exercise the full authority granted to my agent under this power, if my agent, in my agent's sole judgment, determines that the exercise of such authority is appropriate.

9. This power of attorney creates rights only. It does not create any obligation upon my agent to act. My agent shall not incur any liability to me or to anyone claiming through me for acting or refraining from acting under this power of attorney for any action or omission taken in good faith pursuant to this Durable Power of Attorney for Health Care; nor shall my agent be responsible for the actions of any other agent who may have earlier served as my agent.

10. An individual shall be deemed to be unable or unwilling to serve or continue serving as an agent hereunder if: (1) such individual dies, is adjudicated incompetent by a court of competent jurisdiction, or notifies me, the agent(s) serving hereunder, and any successor agent(s) named herein in writing of his/her inability or unwillingness to serve or continue serving as an agent hereunder; (2) two licensed medical doctors who are familiar with the physical and mental condition of such individual determine in a written instrument, a copy of which shall be delivered to me, to the agent(s) serving hereunder, and to any successor

agent(s) named herein, that such individual at the time in question is unable or unwilling to serve or continue serving as such agent; or (3) a court having the requisite jurisdiction determines for any reason that such individual is unable or unwilling to serve or continue serving as such agent.

11. An individual shall be deemed to be unable or unwilling to serve or continue serving as a guardian hereunder if: (1) such individual dies, is adjudicated incompetent by a court of competent jurisdiction, or notifies me, the agent(s) serving hereunder, and any successor guardian(s) named herein in writing of his/her inability or unwillingness to serve or continue serving as a guardian hereunder; (2) two licensed medical doctors who are familiar with the physical and mental condition of such individual determine in a written instrument, a copy of which shall be delivered to me, to the agent(s) serving hereunder, and to any successor guardian(s) named herein, that such individual at the time in question is unable or unwilling to serve or continue serving as such guardian; or (3) a court having the requisite jurisdiction determines for any reason that such individual is unable or unwilling to serve or continue serving as such guardian.

12. I intend this Durable Power of Attorney for Health Care to be exercisable in any state or jurisdiction where I may be at the time in question.

13. I am fully informed as to all the contents of this Durable Attorney for Health Care and understand the full import of this grant of powers to my agent.

Signed:_____(SEAL)

     JANE DOE
     Principal

JANE DOE, the principal, has had an opportunity to read the above Durable Power of Attorney for Health Care and has signed said document in our presence. We, the undersigned, each being over eighteen (18) years of age, hereby witness the principal's signature at the request and in the presence of the principal, and in the presence of each other, the day and year above set out. We further declare that we are not related to the principal by blood, marriage or adoption, and, to the best of my knowledge, we are not entitled to any part of the estate of the principal under a currently existing will or by operation of law, we are not the attending physician of the principal or an employee of a health care facility in which the principal is a patient, nor do we have a claim against the principal or the principal's estate now or after the principal's death.

     Witnesses: Addresses:

_____(Signature)_____

_____(Print Name)_____

_____(Signature)_____

_____(Print Name)_____

STATE OF   §§
COUNTY OF   §

BEFORE ME, the undersigned authority, person-ally appeared JANE DOE to me well known or producing _____ as identification, being by me first duly sworn, who deposes and says that she executed the above and foregoing Durable Power of Attorney for Property for the uses and purposes therein expressed.

WITNESS my hand and seal at the City of _____ , County of _____ , State of _____ , on this _____ day of _____ , 20___.

Notary Public

My Commission Expires:

YOU MAY, BUT ARE NOT REQUIRED TO, REQUEST YOUR AGENT AND SUCCESSOR AGENTS TO PROVIDE SPECIMEN SIGNATURES BELOW. IF YOU INCLUDE SPECIMEN SIGNATURES IN THIS POWER OF ATTORNEY, YOU MUST COMPLETE THE CERTIFICATION OPPOSITE THE SIGNATURES OF THE AGENTS.

Specimen signature of agent (and successor(s)):
_____ AGENT

Agent

_____

SUCCESSOR AGENT

Successor Agent

_____

SUCCESSOR AGENT

Successor Agent

I certify that the signature of my agent (and successor(s)) is correct:

_____
JANE DOE
Principal

_____
JANE DOE
Principal

_____
JANE DOE
Principal

EXAMPLE   **LIVING WILL OF JANE DOE**

If I am not able to make an informed decision regarding my health care, I direct my health care providers to follow my instructions as set forth below. (Initial those statements you wish to be included in the document and cross through those statements which do not apply.)

1. If my death from a terminal condition is imminent and even if life-sustaining procedures are used there is no reasonable expectation of my recovery:

_____   I direct that my life not be extended by life-sustaining procedures, including the administration of nutrition and hydration artificially.

_____ I direct that my life not be extended by life-sustaining procedures, except that, if I am unable to take food by mouth, I wish to receive nutrition and hydration artificially.

_____ I direct that, even in a terminal condition, I be given all available medical treatment in accordance with accepted health care standards.

2. If I am in a persistent vegetative state, that is if I am not conscious and am neither aware of my environment nor able to interact with others, and there is no reasonable expectation of my recovery within a medically appropriate period:

_____ I direct that my life not be extended by life-sustaining procedures, including the administration of nutrition and hydration artificially.

_____ I direct that my life not be extended by life-sustaining procedures, except that if I am unable to take in food by mouth, I wish to receive nutrition and hydration artificially.

_____ I direct that I be given all available medical treatment in accordance with accepted health care standards.

By signing below, I indicate that I am emotionally and mentally competent to make this Living Will and that I understand its purpose and effect.

_____   _____
(Date)   JANE DOE

Declarant
The Declarant signed or acknowledged signing this Living Will in my presence and based upon my personal observation the Declarant appears to be a competent individual.

_____   _____
(Witness)   (Witness)

5. Aphasia/Language Deficits

If your loved one has difficulty communicating with language (as described briefly in chapter 2), their doctor may diagnose primary or secondary aphasia. Aphasia is a group of language deficits that impair language ability. These language deficits can include producing and understanding language: difficulty with reading, writing, and speaking. The causes of aphasia vary from head injury or stroke—in which case the symptoms usually develop with rapid onset—to infection or dementia or learning disability, in which case the symptoms usually develop gradually.

The symptoms and types of aphasia are determined by the area of the brain affected. Some types of aphasia include Broca's aphasia, non-fluent aphasia, motor aphasia, expressive aphasia, receptive aphasia, and global aphasia. Many types of aphasia are treatable while many types of aphasia do not respond to treatment.

Types of Aphasia: Fluent, Non-Fluent and "Pure" Aphasias

Often with fluent aphasia (receptive aphasia), common impairments consist of word repetition or auditory word or phrase or sentence repetition. Impairments with fluent aphasia are related mostly to the input or reception of language. Examples of fluent aphasias are: Wernicke's aphasia, conduction aphasia, anomic aphasia, transcortical motor aphasia, and subcortical aphasia.

Non-fluent aphasias (expressive aphasias) present difficulties in production, but often there is relatively good auditory verbal comprehension. Examples of non-fluent aphasias are: Broca's aphasia, transcortical motor aphasia, and global aphasia.

"Pure" aphasias present impairments in writing, reading, or the recognition of words. These disorders may be idiosyncratic. For example, a person may able to read without problems but have difficulty writing, or is able to write normally but will have difficulty with reading. Examples of pure aphasias are: pure alexia, agraphia, and pure word deafness.

Isolation Aphasia

Another type of language difficulty is isolation aphasia, which is a type of disturbance in communication production, with subsequent effects on the patient's capacity to comprehend what he has heard and acquire new vocabulary. Brain damage, including dementia, can cause this type of aphasia by isolating the speech producing and comprehension cortical structures from each other in the brain.

Symptoms of Aphasia

Symptomology will vary greatly from patient to patient, depending on the causes and progression of the clinical picture. However, the following are some general language impairments common to several forms of aphasia (Alzheimer's Association, 2012; Dementia Guide, 2011; Lewy Body Dementia Association, 2010; Mayo Clinic, 2010; National Institute on Aging, 2011).

- Language impairment in both comprehension and production
- Difficulty with enunciation of words

- Difficulty producing speech
- Difficulty or inability speaking spontaneously
- Difficulty with formation of words
- Difficulty with naming objects
- Difficulty remembering names of people, objects, general categories
- Use of made-up words
- Difficulty repeating a phrase
- Persistent repetition of words or phrases
- Unintentional substitution of letters, syllables, or words
- Difficulty speaking in a grammatically correct way
- Inappropriate use of alterations in inflexion, stress, and rhythm
- Difficulty completing sentences or use of incomplete sentences
- Difficulty reading
- Difficulty writing
- Difficulty creating verbal content

Conduction Aphasia

With conduction aphasia, the patient's ability to comprehend and produce verbal language is often left intact while repetition ability is poor. Conduction aphasia is the result of damage to the cortical structures responsible for production and comprehension of speech. However, it is not clear if this is the only cause of conduction aphasia, as similar symptomology can result from impairment to other cortical structures (Alzheimer's Association, 2012; Dementia Guide, 2011; Lewy Body Dementia Association, 2010; Mayo Clinic, 2010; National Institute on Aging, 2011).

Anomic Aphasia

Patients suffering from anomic aphasia experience profound impairment with naming. This impairment is with naming individual objects and identifying names of whole categories. For example, the patient may have difficulty naming certain people or friends, or they may have difficulty identifying all their daughters as in fact their daughters (or are even people). Anomic aphasia consists mainly with difficulty in naming (Alzheimer's Association, 2012; Dementia Guide, 2011; Lewy Body Dementia Association, 2010; Mayo Clinic, 2010; National Institute on Aging, 2011).

Wernicke's Aphasia

Wernicke's aphasia causes the sufferer to produce long, ongoing sentences that have no meaning, to speak with words that have no meaning, and even create new "words": neologisms. For example, someone with Wernicke's aphasia may say, "You know the cwocker hacked and that I have been here and now and you have it for him," meaning "The cat needs to eat so I will get her food and feed her." Poor auditory and reading comprehension is also a symptom of Wernicke's aphasia, and fluent, but nonsensical, oral and written expression as well. Usually individuals with Wernicke's aphasia have poor insight into their word production errors because they do not comprehend any language, neither their own nor others' (Alzheimer's Association, 2012; Dementia Guide, 2011; Lewy Body Dementia Association, 2010; Mayo Clinic, 2010; National Institute on Aging, 2011).

Broca's Aphasia

Speech produced by patients with Broca's aphasia is usually produced with tremendous effort. It is common for the speaker to produce sentences without words like *is, the,* or *and*. For example, a person with Broca's aphasia may say, "Eat lunch," which could mean "I would like to eat my lunch now, please. Would you please help me prepare my lunch?" or even "Would you like to stay and eat lunch with me today?" It could also mean "I am not interested in eating lunch right now; could we wait until later for lunch, please?" Individuals with Broca's aphasia usually have good insight into their impairment because they are able to understand others' speech to varying degrees. This can often produce frustration as a result of their inability to communicate with others (Alzheimer's Association, 2012; Dementia Guide, 2011; Lewy Body Dementia Association, 2010; Mayo Clinic, 2010; National Institute on Aging, 2011).

Transcortical Motor Aphasia

Transcortical aphasia can present similarly to Broca's aphasia, with speech production coming with tremendous effort from the patient. The speech is often produced with the use of only verbs and nouns. And the patient often retains insight of their impairment. The patient's impairment to comprehend language can deteriorate rapidly as the conversation becomes more complex (Alzheimer's Association, 2012; Dementia Guide, 2011; Lewy Body Dementia Association, 2010; Mayo Clinic, 2010; National Institute on Aging, 2011).

Global Aphasia

Global aphasia can be extremely debilitating for both the speaker and the listener. Individuals with global aphasia have severe communication impairments and will be extremely limited in their ability to produce and comprehend language. Their ability to communicate both verbally and nonverbally can be up to

100 percent impaired. They may have partial ability in some areas or use only nonverbal communication (Alzheimer's Association, 2012; Dementia Guide, 2011; Lewy Body Dementia Association, 2010; Mayo Clinic, 2010; National Institute on Aging, 2011).

Subcortical Aphasias

Symptoms of subcortical aphasia are idiosyncratic as to where and how the specific dementia occurs and in which cortical structures. Symptoms of subcortical aphasia include incomprehensible speech, which appears to make sense to the speakers. Speech seems fluent and effortless and grammatically correct, with impairment in selection of nouns that are replaced with sounds that are not words (or using outright neologisms), and may perseverate (or repeat at length) if they try to replace the words they can't find with sounds (Alzheimer's Association, 2012; Dementia Guide, 2011; Lewy Body Dementia Association, 2010; Mayo Clinic, 2010; National Institute on Aging, 2011).

Clinical Case Example of Lara:

Lara is an eighty-one-year-old African-American woman who lives alone in a single-family home in rural northern America. She has lived independently since her husband passed away fifteen years ago. Lara has no living children. Lara lives with a twenty-four-hour live-in staff provided by a home care agency that provides all of her personal care and arranges for all of her medical and psychiatric care. Lara is in good general physical health, has had a hip replacement within the last two years due to a fall, and has a recurring UTI (urinary tract infection). She takes an antidepressant medication for sleep, which is helpful, and a neuroleptic for aggressive behaviors, which is also helpful.

Lara has profound global aphasia, and it is therefore difficult to accurately assess most of her other symptoms of dementia. Her language is sometimes 80 percent impaired and at other times, it is sometimes 100 percent impaired. Additionally, she confabulates—this is when the patient has some sense of a memory or understanding of reality but there are gaps, so they fill those gaps in with something they think makes sense, using environmental cues and pieces of other memories accessible at the moment.

When you are sitting with Lara, she will begin a "conversation" with you without hesitation. Lara has no insight about her language impairment and she expects her conversation to be understood by her listener. Some days this can happen because there is enough language production that one can carry on by using vague terms and answers to volley banter back and forth. However, most of the time this is not possible, and because of her lack of insight, Lara can become agitated and aggressive as she tries to make sense of why her conversation partner is refusing to talk with her.

Lara's affective communication is still intact, so when she uses her verbal communication skills, as impaired as these might be, there is always a way to tap into the prosody in her voice—and her to tap into the prosody of others'. In other words, you cannot understand what she is saying, but you can usually understand how she is saying it. She is very expressive emotionally, and this is how she communicates most of the time. When she is happy, her voice sounds happy. When she is frightened, her voice sounds frightened, and so forth.

Lara responds positively to nonverbal cues like facial expressions and other body language and tone of voice. She can understand smiling faces and gentle voices, and she will smile back and her face will soften when she hears a calm voice (if it comes from a person who is looking at her). She also responds positively to someone talking to her with their arms physically open and head tilted gently to one side as they speak to her. *Holding hands and hugs are also types of communication she understands.*

Lara has lost her ability to read and write; therefore, using this path of communication is not an option. Interestingly, she does seem to have insight regarding her loss of reading and writing skills, as measured by her reactions when offered pen and paper or reading material. She will show behavioral signs of embarrassment and anger when offered the option to write her answers on paper, which indicates she is aware she has lost these skills and that something is wrong.

It is difficult to assess a patient with such profound aphasia, because neurophych assessment is usually done with either a conversation or with a pencil and paper. Neither of these options are reliable with a patient with severe language deficits because you will probably be measuring their language impairment rather that other symptoms of dementia. There is always neuro-imaging like functional magnetic resonance imaging (FMRI) and computerized axial tomography (CAT) scans; however, knowing where the damage exists still leaves you to guess what the resulting experience will be exactly like for each individual.

6. How to Communicate with Your Loved One Who Has a Language Deficit

As a progressive illness, one can expect dementia to continue to cause communication to become increasingly difficult for you and your loved one. Communicating basic, everyday facts will eventually become a challenge as names, dates, and places become lost forever. Dementia will gradually affect the way your loved one is able to present rational ideas and their ability to reason clearly will change.

Communicating with your loved one can be challenging because someone with dementia will often feel confused, frightened, angry, or humiliated. Your loved one may resist you or become aggressive when you try to provide personal care such as bathing or feeding. The person who is confused may ask about loved ones who are no longer living, repeat himself over and over, or may not be able to speak at all. There are some helpful strategies that seem to facilitate communication universally. Then there are some ways in which your loved one will need his own particular type of assistance that you will need to figure out together as you go along.

Communication is a complicated, two-way process. Not only is it important that your loved one is encouraged to use whatever different skills, verbal and nonverbal, are necessary to communicate, but also you as a caregiver may have to learn to listen differently.

Try to become attuned to your loved one as they communicate with you. Pay attention to the way their facial expressions change and the way their emotional content in their voice changes. The loudness and softness of their voice is communication; the way they use their body has meaning as well as the actual words they say. Now you can be attuned to them by mirroring their nonverbal cues. Did they smile as they spoke? Then you smile back, because whatever they were communicating to you, it contained emotional content that required a smile. If you return this similar facial expression, then you are telling them that you "got it."

Prepare to be frustrated and at times confused. Don't hesitate to walk away when the "conversation" begins to go nowhere. Come back and try again a few minutes later. The following are some general strategies to consider regarding communication with your loved one suffering from dementia.

Think about your body language. Use your posture, facial expressions, voice, and physical proximity to communicate, as well as your words. Display a calm and gentle manner. Your demeanor communicates how you are feeling to your loved one: when you look calm and gentle your loved one will feel this from you.

Try not to use negative words such as "don't do that" or "stop doing that." Negative language can cause feelings of shame for people who are already struggling; try to frame requests in positive ways. For example, rather than saying "Don't put your shoes over there," try asking "Please put your shoes over here."

Try to use questions that utilize cues rather than short-term memory alone, such as "What did you have for lunch today?" Using short, simple instructions is more helpful. Try asking "Did you enjoy your lunch today?" Utilize your loved one's long-term memory, such as "I hear you were a wonderful cook when you were young."

Try to encourage your loved one to engage the conversation by making it easy. Trying to iron out too many details can be confusing to your loved one, and asking them to repeat themselves might require too much short-term memory, which can be confusing and frustrating. Avoid arguing and ordering the person around; being patient and remaining calm can help the person communicate more easily. Using a positive and friendly tone of voice whenever possible is also a means of effective communication.

Be mindful of personal space with your loved one during interactions. Standing in someone's personal space can feel intimidating or threatening; alternatively, not engaging the person by standing too far away can give the impression that you are aloof or uninterested in them. Do not be afraid to touch your loved in appropriate ways. Holding their hand or patting them on the arm can contribute significantly to the quality of your interactions and make them feel cared for. Making consistent eye contact with the person you talk to shows them you are interested in what they are saying and that you are paying attention to them.

Move slowly through the conversation with your loved one, and allow them enough time to respond to your questions. Engage them with eye contact and facial expressions that show them you would like to talk with them. Although it may be tempting at times, try not to finish their sentences or answer questions that others have asked them. This might give them the impression that you believe they cannot answer for himself, and create feelings of anger and shame.

When your loved one seems confused or cannot speak directly to the content of the conversation, try not to dismiss what they have said. They are still contributing to the conversation, and this is meaningful to them. Rather, try to add to their contribution without pointing out that they may have strayed off topic. Encourage them to continue with the conversation by making it easy for them to follow along, and show them you value their contributions.

Your loved one may need more time to express himself; allow them ample time to say everything they are trying to say. Resist the temptation to interrupt, even if you think you already know what they are going to say.

Keep the area you occupy while communicating with your loved one free of distractions like televisions and radios and extraneous conversations. Try not to multitask while communicating with your loved one; give them your undivided attention. Try not to confuse them with too many choices or a conversation that is too complicated. Avoid asking them too many questions during the conversation.

Listening in a Different Way

Examine your loved one's body language for clues about what they are trying to communicate to you. Stomping a foot or frowns are signs of disapproval or distress or anger. Scan the environment to identify why your loved one may be showing signs of being unhappy, and try to connect their feelings to their environment. Then ask short pointed yes/no questions that are very specific to the indicated distress. For example, if your loved one is eating and stomping their foot, you might ask if they like this food. Depending on which direction they shake their head, your next question might be whether they would like a different type of food or if they are finished eating or if they don't feel well.

Try not to assume you understand your loved one's body language correctly. Repeat back to them what you think they are telling you, and then ask, "Did I understand you correctly?'" If you get a negative response, try again to figure out what they are trying to tell you.

While you wait for your loved one to respond, try to wait patiently. Be mindful of your posture, your facial expressions, and any other gestures you might be making with your body. Try to create a peaceful atmosphere for your loved one while they express himself and puts words to their experience.

When you are having difficulty understanding your loved one, let them know. Try saying, "I am having a hard time understand you right now." Try not to blame the person, and if they become frustrated, then take a little break from the conversation and come back to it later. Be certain to assure the person that you intend to return to the conversation so they don't feel dismissed, but if they don't remember about it later, it might be a good idea to just let it go.

Observe Nonverbal Communication

Only about 10 percent of our communication is comprised of words, while the rest of what we communicate comes from nonverbal sources. Therefore, when you have a loved one with language deficits, there is a lot you can do to communicate that does not involve language. For example, if your loved one can gesture or point, then try to recognize what they are attempting to tell you and encourage this interaction and use of communication. People who have aphasia may be tempted to withdraw from others and may be at high risk for depression and isolation due to their inability to communicate. Therefore, any way you can help them communicate can be helpful to them for many reasons.

If your loved one is unable to speak answers to your questions but is capable of understanding your questions, then ask them short, simple questions that can be answered with yes/no answers. Determine with them one gesture for *yes* and one gesture for *no*: for example, a head shake in one direction for *yes* and a head shake in another direction for *no*. Ask more questions to collect details but only one detail at a time.

Use Communication Boards

A communication board can be a simple homemade board or a complex, costly store-bought board. You can use dry-erase boards, pen and paper for writing messages, alphabet letters to arrange on a board, or something pre-made with words your loved one can point to. The message board is anything that can be used in which you can communicate back and forth using messages left for each other.

Focus on Abilities of the Person with Dementia

Your loved one will probably lose their short-term memory ability before they lose their crystallized long-term memory. This memory impairment will be noticeable and limiting in functioning as well as frustrating for both you and your loved one. However, there are ways to make the most of your loved one's strengths without overtaxing their abilities. Here are some suggestions:

- Encourage your loved one to re-live and reminisce their crystallized memories
- Provide encouragement for a job well done and positive effort

- Provide reassurance for times that become challenging and stressful
- Provide enough time for processing to prevent the person from becoming confused or disoriented
- Understand your loved one may be experiencing memories in pieces and may be unable to recall complete facts
- Encourage independence by allowing the person to do what he can for himself and assist with the rest

It can be challenging not to react to your loved one in a negative way when they are acting aggressively or hostile. Without realizing, you might talk about your loved one as though they are not present, but this can foster an environment of disrespect or dismissiveness for your loved one, leaving them feeling shamed or angry.

Treat your loved one with dignity and respect regardless of their behavior. If you need to walk away for a moment to calm down yourself, by all means do that. Secure the area for your loved one so they are safe, and then take a "time-out" for yourself.

Avoid treating your loved one like a child. Although they might not be able to make well-thought-out decisions, they are still an adult with adult feelings and can experience shame, guilt, and anger when treated with disrespect or dismissed. Never speak in the person's presence as if they are not there—discuss care issues somewhere private where they can't hear you.

Encourage independence according to your loved one's abilities. Try to look for places where your loved one can succeed and celebrate that with them rather than focusing on where they need more help.

Communicating with a loved one who has dementia can be quite challenging, but you can be creative and have fun with your loved one to foster more effective communication. By focusing on respect, nonverbal cues, and meeting your loved one's needs based on his existing abilities, you may enhance communication with someone who is confused.

Clinical Case Example of Lucy

Lucy is a seventy-three-year-old Asian woman who lives with her with two daughters in a large home in a rural community. Lucy is in good health and suffers from moderate dementia with mild memory loss. She becomes confused about time and dates and can forget where she is and the purpose of her visits. She experiences personality and mood changes and suffers from agitation and paranoia, which causes her to withdraw from family members and isolate herself sometimes. These feelings impair her ability to communicate with others because she, at times fears that people are trying to harm her or steal things from her; her reaction to this is to become aggressive. Lucy also experiences mild productive aphasia, causing her to have difficulty speaking, while her ability to understand what others say to her is intact.

Upon first meeting Lucy, she appears gentle and somewhat docile, with a small build and passive demeanor. Lucy looks away when she speaks and doesn't look her conversation partner in the eye. As the conversation progresses and the details become more taxing, it becomes easier to see that Lucy is not following the conversation. She will use strategies like nodding her head or looking away to avoid making it clear that she has lost her way in the conversation. At times, she will resort to aggression to take the focus off her communication impairment.

Rather than pointing out to Lucy that I have noticed that she has lost her place in the conversation, because this will cause shame for her, I pace myself with her. As she is unable to keep up, I just let go of the conversation also. I wait a minute or so, and begin a new but related topic of conversation with enough context that Lucy can follow along. For example, when we were talking about her daughter's cat, she said, "This is Tabby she's my daughter's cow." I said, "Your daughter's cat is lovely, how long have you had her?' but Lucy did not respond to this question; she continued to pet the cat. So I pet the cat as well and after about a minute, I said, "This is a lovely cat, I have a cat at home myself." Then Lucy said, "This is my daughter's cow. What is your cow's name?" I responded, "her name is Maria and she looks a lot like this one here." In this way, we could continue a conversation without frustration or embarrassment to Lucy for not being able to follow along.

7. Managing Your Loved One's Problem Behaviors

Different people suffer from behavior problems in different ways when dementia is concerned. One person might never experience a disturbance in sleep architecture while someone else might experience wandering throughout the night or sun downing problems. Listed here is a generic description of some behaviors that can become problematic for some people, and when they do become problematic, they present differently for most people and in different combinations.

Wandering

Your loved one may wander in an attempt to fulfill many different needs that they may not be able to articulate; for example, they may become disinterested in their environment, they may be experiencing medication side effects and cannot express their physical discomfort, they may be experiencing pain, or they may be looking for something or someone. Perhaps their wandering is due to an unfulfilled biological need like hunger or thirst, or they might need to use the bathroom. They might simply have a natural need for exercise or movement and be trying to get a stretch or some exercise in. Wandering does have its inherent problems; your loved one might wander out into the night, or they could just wander off and get lost or injured.

If you are concerned about your loved one's wandering, there are things you can do to protect them; for example, consider installing locks that are too high up or too complicated for your loved one to unlock by himself, or consider installing a lock that requires a key to unlock or one that requires a code. People with dementia can become confused easily, so if you place a curtain over the door, this may distract your loved one from opening the door. Consider using a black cardboard shape like a circle over the floor in front of the door. This might confuse your loved one and look like a hole in the floor and they will not walk over the "hole" in the floor to get out of the door. Using child-safety devices are helpful. You can obtain child-safety devices that fit over door-knobs to prevent children from opening doors.

Arrange a meeting with neighbors and friends to alert them about your loved one's tendency to wander and ask them to let you know if they should see your loved one outside without you. Make sure your neighbors and friends have a current contact number for you, and ask them to call the local police department if you are unavailable when they call. Home security systems are available to fit most budgets; they can be helpful when your loved one opens a window or door without turning off the security alarm system. Your loved one can carry digital devices that use a global positioning system, so if they should become lost your local police department will be able to locate them. This could be worn as a bracelet or a necklace. There are many different styles of identification necklaces and bracelets available that you might think about for your loved one.

Incontinence

Incontinence may become a problem for your loved one at some point, and accidents may happen due to loss of bladder or bowel control. Confusion may also contribute when they forget or cannot figure out where the bathroom is or how to navigate the toilet, or it might just take too long to remember all these things. Try not to shame your loved one around toileting issues because these are private and, for most, sensitive issues. For most people, needing assistance using the toilet can be humiliating, and even the slightest perception of disrespect can cause feelings of shame and anger and will be emotionally wounding for your loved one.

Expect accidents to happen, but try to not make a big deal about it; best case will be to avoid accidents and help your loved one to succeed in this area. Consider using tape on the floor, marking a trail to the bathroom, or using signs on the bathroom door, marking the room so your loved one will know which room is the bathroom in case they forget. Establish a routine for using the toilet. Use the same bathroom schedule every day and help your loved one with it. For example, take your loved one to the bathroom every three hours and go through the bathroom ritual with them.

Limit the amount of liquids you allow your loved one to consume in the evenings, and try to encourage her to drink most liquids in the daytime. Be mindful of the types of liquids you are using, and avoid caffeinated beverages and alcohol. Consider getting a bedside commode from a medical supply store for your loved one's bedside for overnights or when she's napping. Use incontinence pads and products, which can be purchased from a medical supply store and many grocery stores, for both your loved one and their bed. Think about applying Velcro strips to the clothing for quick and easy removal should an accident occur during the night.

Agitation

Agitation occurs on a continuum, with agitation and irritability on the lower end, hostility and violence on the upper end, and aggression (both verbal and physical) about in the middle. You will see an increase in these symptoms as your loved one's illness

81

progresses. Agitation can occur as your loved one experiences increased loss of their independence and realizes they depend more and more on family, friends, and strangers for needs they were once able to fulfill himself.

Consider reducing or eliminating the caffeine and alcohol your loved one takes. Environmental factors can contribute to agitation; for example, too much noise or too many distractions can cause your loved one to be overwhelmed and agitated. Try using cues like photographs or familiar objects when your loved one is in an unfamiliar place, to decrease the level of extraneous distractions.

When your loved one becomes agitated, try holding their hand or touching their arm; sometimes using soft, soothing music can be helpful. Do not try to speak louder than they are speaking; the calmness and gentleness in your voice will be soothing. If you are attempting to use physical restraints, expect increased physical violence because putting on restraints will cause panic: your loved one might not understand why you are restraining him; they might think you are attacking them and try to protect himself. Keep the environment safe for your loved one and remove any dangerous objects so they do not reach for anything while agitated.

Agitation and anxiety are interrelated. Any type of highly emotionally charged encounter can elevate anxiety for your loved one, and, because anxiety is interrelated with the agitation continuum, this emotional encounter becomes a negative feedback loop: anxiety increases agitation, which increases anxiety, which further increases agitation, and so on. Your loved one can be easily distracted, so try intervening with a different and interesting activity like offering a snack or carrying the family pet. Think of how your loved one can use their independence in the situation, then make their independent action the central focus of the interaction; this will help her feel in control, thus decreasing her agitation and increasing their feelings of competence and confidence and happiness.

Sleeplessness and Sun Downing

Agitation, confusion, disorientation, restlessness, and isolation often get worse at the end of the day and often continue throughout the night. This pattern of behavior is common to patients suffering from dementia. This is a complex behavior caused by many factors including exhaustion and confusion in the patient's biological clock and circadian rhythms. Discouraging napping during the daytime can be helpful, as can encouraging daytime activities and exercise. Also try limiting caffeine, sugar, and alcoholic beverages, and coordinating meals into three small meals (with no meals too close to bedtime). Late afternoon walks or listening to music before bedtime can also be helpful. During sunset, close the curtains and turn on extra lights to minimize the effect of the ambient environment. Use a night-light near the stairways and in bathrooms, or use a gate to prevent falls at dangerous places in the house. There are medications that assist with relaxation and sleep that might be appropriate for your loved one.

Bathing

Bathing can be a challenge for people with dementia. Bathing can be a private experience for most people because when we bathe, we are undressed and cleaned. Even when someone we love and trust is helping, it can still be a humiliating experience. When we are bathing we are exposed and vulnerable, and if we become confused it can be a frightening experience. Therefore, bathing can be a source of extreme distress for someone who is suffering from dementia.

When you are helping your loved one bathe, think of their historical hygiene routine. Did they take baths or showers? Were these in the morning or at night? Did they go to the beautician to have their hair washed, or did they do it himself? Did they use lotions, powders, bubbles, scents, or did they use only soap and water? If your loved one has lived their life as a modest individual, continue with this.

Turn your head as much as you can without putting their in danger. Try to keep the doors closed, but stay inside the bathroom with them. Keep a towel up and available for them to cover as much of their body as they wish, and lift the towel as you ash each area of their body. Let them participate in selecting their robe or clothing they will put on after their bath, and have the clothing ready and close to the tub so you can help them get dressed directly after her bath. Always have towels and a robe nearby and ready immediately when your loved one gets out of the shower or tub.

Elderly people are more sensitive to both hot and cold, so make sure the temperature of the water and the temperature in the room are comfortable for them. Your loved one might be afraid of falling, so use bath mats with non-slip grips, hand railings, and a shower seat to make your loved one feel safe. Make sure you bring everything you will need with you, because you should never leave a person with dementia unattended in the bath or shower. Older people are often afraid of falling, so help them feel secure.

Apathy

Apathy can include behaviors like lack of motivation, listlessness, and passive attitudes and behaviors, which can lead to isolation and social withdrawal. This can become a problem with a person suffering from dementia because this causes their world to eventually become smaller and smaller, until there is nothing left but her own house.

Staying active increases your loved one's physical health and wards off depression. Apathy can be a symptom of certain other health conditions as well as depression, so be sure to report signs of apathy to her physician. Try engaging them in enjoyable activities, but construct these activities to something she can enjoy and modify them so they can have some degree of autonomy while participating. Anything your loved one can do will be helpful to them.

Use your own enthusiasm to her them interested; if you are enjoying an activity, then it must be worth doing. Try small steps; if you can get them interested in holding some hairbrushes and barrettes, then it will be easier to get them to let you brush their hair.

Confusion

Confusion is common with dementia. Your loved one may become confused about who they are, who others are, or where they are, or confused about the time or date or even the year. Confusion can also occur regarding why things are happening and why your loved one is doing something. This confusion may be present in one situation while at another time, even in the same situation, your loved one may be completely lucid. Confusion about the purpose of objects is also common. For example, your loved one might try to use a drinking glass for a telephone or try to use a shoe for a television's remote control.

Try to stay calm and provide simple, clear, positive feedback when you are asked for help. If you are not asked for help, and your loved one is not hurting himself or anyone else, you might just let them go ahead and talk on the drinking glass or point the shoe at the television. But keep an eye on him and intervene when they are in trouble. When they is trying to eat and can't identify his spoon, for example, you might say, "Here is your spoon, and it's for eating your food." You might coach them how to use a spoon by using your own spoon. Never shame them for misusing objects (or not knowing something you think he should know or something he knew yesterday).

Repetition

Repetition is a behavior of people with dementia: they might repeat a sound, word, question, or action again and again. This usually occurs in the middle to late stages of the disease, and indicates your loved one is feeling insecure or fearful. Engaging in repetition might comfort them when they are feeling out of control. While this is usually harmless, it can be extremely unnerving for caregivers.

Consider the comforting benefit of the repetitive behavior and if the discomfort it responds to has an environmental source, an emotional source, or perhaps both. Try to figure out what the behavior is accomplishing for the person. This will increase the likelihood of responding in a way that will benefit your loved one. If the repetitive behavior in something other than speech, try using it in a way your loved one can feel useful and helpful. For example, if your loved one is constantly moving objects around, try giving them some laundry to sort or some books to put away.

Suspicion

People with dementia can become suspicious of others, and they can become suspicious of you as well. It's common for them to make accusations of all kinds of things ranging from theft to infidelity. Try to remember what dementia symptoms are about, and try not to be offended. Don't try to convince your loved one that you are innocent, because this might increase their suspicion. Try to answer with something simple like "I see you are very upset about that" or "I will try my best to help you with that."

Storing extra items that are frequently lost can be helpful. For example, if your loved one often loses her coin purse, having an extra similar coin purse to bring out can be helpful. Redirecting at this time can also help alleviate her anxiety:. suggest having a bowl of ice cream, for example, or pick up the house cat and offer for her to pet it.

Clinical Case Example of Leonard

Leonard is an eighty-two-year-old Italian American man who has a large family and many friends. He spent most of his life living with his wife, who passed away two years ago, at which time he began living with his oldest son. Leonard has always been a happy, friendly, and social person who was well loved by most people who knew him.

Leonard started becoming irritable with family members about three years ago, prior to his diagnosis of dementia. His irritability sometimes escalated to agitation and left friends and family members confused because this behavior was uncharacteristic. For example, while watching television, without warning he might just jump up and storm out of the room, or in a conversation he might go from a friendly banter to sudden rage and accusations of others' lying or trying to bully him. He also started to hoard things of no apparent value in his garage at home. He became very stingy with other things of value like money, and he no longer allowed family members to use his personal items like his cars, although he was once a very generous person. At times, Leonard tried to start arguments with people in public whom he did not know, as though he was defending himself from perceived insult.

Upon first meeting Leonard, the impression I got was that he was a genuinely kind and social person. He seemed to enjoy my company and was easy to engage in conversation. But as we continued to talk, it became noticeable that he was having an internal experience that was different from mine. For example, I began conducting a standard clinical interview, which consists of the same questions I ask most patients, like questions about age, a few demographic questions, and a few open-ended questions about symptomology. Within the first few questions, Leonard became somewhat aggressive and demanded to know why I wanted to know about his "personal business" and why I was so being "nosey." I quickly changed my strategy and, to avoid confrontation by frightening him, invited him to tell me what he wanted me to know about himself. Leonard was unable to put all the pieces together—that I was asking these questions because I was his doctor—and this left him to try to make sense of the situation. Because he was already suspicious, he thought I was being nosey. By giving the control back to him, since he trusts himself, I avoided the risk of his suspicion escalating into paranoia.

Paranoia can be like a delusion, and when someone believes you are trying to harm him, the more you try to convince him you are not going to harm him, the more you are actually convincing him he's right in thinking he can't trust you. According to his paranoid thinking, if he could trust you, then you would agree with him. Agreeing with a suspicious and paranoid person who does not trust you means you agree that you are not a safe person, and you're then colluding with his delusion that you mean to cause harm.

This was part of the problem with Leonard's family. They did not understand what was going on with Leonard, especially prior to his diagnosis of dementia. Naturally, they were trying to talk about his behavior and feelings like they would with any other person who was not experiencing dementia or paranoia. In some ways, this made the experience worse, which led to more confusion and hurt feelings.

Leonard only reacted with suspicion and agitation sometimes because he processed information in his brain differently at different times. As his dementia progresses, his presentation will change. This is good news because there are many times when Leonard is not suspicious or paranoid—but in some ways, this is confusing for those around him. It can be difficult to understand why someone with dementia has what doctors call a punctuated presentation of symptomology. People with other illnesses have their symptoms all the time, right? But dementia is different. Leonard and many others have good days and bad days when their symptoms are better or worse.

Hallucinations

Your loved one may experience hallucinations and delusions, which might be frightening and cause significant distress. Hallucinations can be either visual (when they see things that are not really there) or audio (when they hear things that are not really there). It is possible to have other sensory perceptions as hallucinations—to hallucinate how things feel, smell, or taste—but it is far less common. Delusions are strong beliefs about things that are not really happening: for example, they might believe a loved one who has died is not really dead, or that people are stealing from them, or that they have another home to go to.

When your loved one is experiencing a hallucination or delusion, do not try to convince them that the experience is not real. If you try to do this, you run the risk of becoming a part of the experience but in a negative way. For example, if your loved one believes people are stealing from them, and you try to convince them this is not the case, they may become suspicious of you as well in an attempt to make sense of why you do not believe them. It is best to empathize with their feelings without colluding with the belief. For example, you might say something like "Oh, how frightening that must feel, for your things to keep going missing."

Should the hallucinations be of a pleasant nature, then is it really a problem at this point? If you notice your loved one laughing or smiling or chatting pleasantly with someone in the room that you cannot see, maybe that's not such a bad thing. Maybe their internal experience is something they enjoy and this might be something you might want to let them keep for himself.

Hallucinations and delusions can sometimes be managed with medications, and sometimes they cannot. Consult with a board-certified psychiatrist for a medication consultation to get a proper evaluation for your loved one.

Clinical Case Example of Charlotte

Charlotte is an eighty-four-year old-Caucasian woman who lives alone but with twenty-four-hour in-home care in a single home dwelling in a large city. Charlotte has moderate dementia with severe cognitive deficits, moderate language impairments, and hallucinations. She has difficulty bathing and eating and can be aggressive and violent at times.

Charlotte's cognitive impairments include memory deficits that prevent her from doing things that involve planning, like cooking, shopping, or cleaning house. She is unable to find rooms in her house, and when she goes outside, she is unable to find her way home. When she wakes up at night to go to the bathroom, she often gets lost in her own home. Charlotte's in-home health aides sleep in her room with her in their own bed so that Charlotte will always be able to find them. They also use tape to mark trails in the house for her to follow from room to room. And they supervise her activities for her safety.

Charlotte has an aversion to bathing, and this has become an increasing challenge with the progression of her dementia. Her health aides use several techniques to assist this process. One thing they do that has been helpful is trying to approach Charlotte at different times with the task of bathing. Charlotte will give vastly different responses even a few minutes apart. If Charlotte responds negatively the first time they ask, they just ask a few minutes or an hour later and usually get a different response. Another technique that is effective with Charlotte is draping her body while bathing her. Using a soft, warm towel to cover her body while washing her provides an atmosphere of modesty for her and is very helpful. Her aides uncover only the part of her body that is necessary to wash then cover her back up before proceeding to another part of her body. Providing this modesty for Charlotte is very helpful while bathing her.

Eating is a challenge for Charlotte. Providing delicious and pleasant-looking food is helpful but not sufficient to get Charlotte to eat. Sometimes Charlotte will eat the food on her own if it is interesting and appealing enough, but sometimes she just forgets what to do with the food, and her health aides need to coach her on what to do with the food. Her aides need to take a bite and show her how to take a bite of food, maybe even several times, then Charlotte will start to eat on her own. Sometimes this is not enough and her health aides need to feed her.

When Charlotte becomes aggressive and violent it is best to try to de-escalate only by keeping the environment safe for her and allowing her to have space. The aides show themselves as nonthreatening by way of facial expression and body posture which is the only intervention that is advised when Charlotte is aggressive or violent. If you try to argue or tell her what to do after she becomes aggressive or violent, she will likely escalate and the situation will worsen. However, when using this strategy, it is important to make sure there is nothing in the environment that can hurt her, like something that can be grabbed impulsively to use as a weapon or something she can fall down onto.

8. In-Home Services, Assisted-Living Facilities, Skilled-Nursing Facilities, and Hospitals

Several factors are important to consider when trying to decide which living arrangements are best for your loved one. Consider your options, your budget, and some of your loved one's needs and other ways they can be met. Everyone's situation is unique and dynamic and every situation is different; only you and your loved one can decide which is the best choice for you. Here are some of the issues to consider when evaluating your options.

In-Home Services

Many families and older adults prefer to stay in the comfort if their own home and age in familiar surroundings. But how do you know if this is the right choice for you and your loved one? The goal of in-home care services is to help you remain at home comfortably as long as possible, rather than moving into a long-term care facility. This can be a good choice for individuals who have a strong network of friends and family to help them, viable financial resources, and need only minor assistance with their daily activities.

Your loved one will naturally want to stay in their home as long as possible, and with the assistance of in-home services, they can do just that for longer than without in-home professional help. There are many choices regarding in-home services: explore the options and make informed decisions. Ask friends and health-care providers if they have had experiences with in-home care and get their input.

No doubt, most people would like to continue to live at home as long as they can; this is a natural desire. However, sometimes there are parts of the bigger picture that conflict with this desire. Sudden loss of a support or social network, illness, unforeseen financial difficulties, or a geographical move are examples of factors that may influence an adult's decision to leave home. Too often, decisions to leave home are made suddenly, after your loved one's illness, making adjustments all the more painful and difficult.

Finances

Anticipate which expenses you are likely to incur, and make a budget that includes everything you can think of. Get a good look at your situation. In-home services can be arranged on any budget, but twenty-four-hour coverage can be expensive. You can arrange financial management assistance (see the Resources section at the end of this book) if you're having trouble with managing your or your loved one's finances.

Practical Considerations

Rural areas can be farther away from grocery stores and doctor's offices, and more difficult for relatives and health-care professionals to access, so more time will be spent driving than if your loved one was in a more accessible urban area. If you're in an area with more public transit, community resources might be safe and easily accessible. How much time does it take for your loved one to get to services such as shopping or doctor's appointments?

Your loved one may be struggling with transportation and driving might become a challenge for them. Driving at night or driving at all can be overwhelming for your loved one. Considering transportation options can help you keep them at home and maintain their independence and social network. You may want to consider local transportation such as buses, taxis, and special senior transportation options to travel to appointments. Transportation options are also available through in-home service programs.

You may need to modify your home, so think about how much effort you will be putting into home modifications. Steps and stairs need to be considered, as well as yard work and landscaping. You also might need to install fences, gates, and security alarms to keep your loved one safe at home.

As your loved one's mobility becomes more limited, their needs will require home modifications to accommodate their limited mobility. Around the house your loved one will benefit from modifications like bathroom shower bars and handles, ramps to modify stairs, and possibly renovating the downstairs so they do not have the need to use the stairs at all.

Keeping up with the household chores can be challenging. Consider laundry, shopping, gardening, housekeeping, and handyman services to supplement what you can't keep up with.

There will be times when you cannot leave home for long periods of time due to the care you will be providing for your loved one; without help, isolation can rapidly set in. You may need to give up once-meaningful activities like hobbies, community involvement, or visits with friends and family. Losing these connections and support may lead to your own depression, which will adversely affect both you and your loved one.

Your own health, like having a medical condition that may worsen with stress or just progress with time might make in-home services an especially valuable resource to consider. It's important to think about issues like your own mobility problems, medication issues, and other complications that are likely to result from a medical condition.

Consider how viable your social support is. How nearby are your friends and family, and are they willing to relieve you and help provide the necessary support to your loved one? Many older adults prefer to rely on family to provide help, but as your needs increase, family alone might not be able to fill in all the gaps. Consider community services like churches and community health centers as social support as well.

Adult day programs are helpful for both your loved one and for you, providing entertainment and socialization for your loved one and a respite breaks for you as a caregiver. There are different kinds of adult day programs: while some are social and recreational, others focus on therapeutic value and may specialize in specific disorders such as early stage Alzheimer's.

Having others help you take care of your loved one can be tremendously helpful even if you have strong family support. It is not uncommon to feel like you do not want strangers in your home; many people have this initial feeling, but the benefit of receiving help with caregiving is worth the initial discomfort for most people. Taking care of a loved one with dementia can be exhausting both emotionally and physically, especially if the responsibility is primarily on one person such as a spouse or adult child. Your relationships can be vastly improved if you are open to the idea of receiving assistance from more than one resource.

Custodial care is the assistance of activities of daily living: things like eating, dressing, bathing, and meal preparation. Assistance with these activities can be provided by in-home health aides or personal care aides. In-home health aides and personal care aides might also provide things like shopping, medication reminders, appointment management and reminders, and laundry assistance. The level of care that can be provided by in-home services ranges from only a few hours at a time to twenty-four-hour live-in care.

Often, health-care professionals will make home visits to provide treatment at home. For example, home nurses and hospice workers will come to their patients' homes to provide services. Sometimes your insurance will work with in-home service programs to provide coverage for these services, although you may have to cover some cost out of pocket.

Hiring Home Care Providers

While evaluating home care services, try to obtain referrals from as many different sources as possible. When considering a provider, here are some issues to think about:

Benefits of home care agencies include the dependability of knowing they have prescreened their care providers as well as knowing back-up care will be provided should your caregiver become ill or otherwise no longer be able to provide care to your loved one. Agencies also have insurance coverage, should something happen to their providers while on the job. However, these benefits come with a price: agencies are usually a lot more expensive than independent providers.

When working with an agency, read your contract carefully and ask questions to clarify anything you might not be clear about. Ask about what the fee covers and when additional fees would be applied. Ask about when the last time rate increases were applied and if they are expecting any increases in the future. Ask about their termination procedures and policies.

You can usually employ independent providers for a significantly lower fee, and you are able to negotiate you own terms of service with them. However, you need to do your own background screening and prearrange for back-up coverage if for some reason the independent provider is unable to come to work.

The way in which you go about hiring home care providers will depend on what kind of help you are looking for. Should you be considering hiring someone to help with shopping or household maintenance, you would be exploring different options than if you were considering hiring someone to provide in-home care for your loved one. Something to keep in mind that is usually true is that spending as much time as possible with your candidate will help you make a well-informed decision regarding the hiring process. Explore as many options as possible while hiring a provider. Conduct as many hiring interviews as possible before making a decision. When meeting a candidate for the first time, try to meet them in a public place where there are other people, even if they have been referred to you from someone you know or an agency.

When checking references, examine for where references are provided from; they should come from more than one source. Look for unexplained gaps in histories from references. When talking with referred candidates, listen to their tone, and listen both to what they do say and what they do not say. Are they happy to provide a reference for the person or do they seem less than enthusiastic with short answers to your question?

When conducting background checks, make sure to do background checks on every candidate you are considering for employment. Unless you're working through an agency, you'll need to do the background checks yourself. You can use the

Internet or your local police department, legal aid service, or use an attorney for referrals to individuals or companies that do background checks on individuals for private employment.

If you feel uncomfortable with a candidate for any reason, do not hesitate to move on to the next person. It's especially important that you feel comfortable with an employee, because this person is providing services for your loved one in your own home. Try talking with the provider for explanations about anything you are unsure of. Sometimes, things you feel uncomfortable about can be worked out. If not, don't be afraid to find another caregiver.

Know what you need from your provider and ask specific question to be sure your provider knows what you are expecting from her. Allow your provider to describer her qualifications in detail and listen for anything that concerns you, then follow-up with more questions. Ask about experience with what you are hiring for and if your provider is comfortable with what you need. Develop a written contract specifically addressing everything you discussed with your provider, and seal it with a signature.

Case Example of Ernie

Ernie is a seventy-six-year-old Latino man who resides alone in a single-family home in a large city. He has lived alone for twenty years, since his wife passed away. Ernie has no children. Ernie has mild dementia with mild cognitive deficits; mild to moderate personality and mood impairment that can include agitation and aggression; and difficulty controlling impulsive behavior, including inappropriate sexual behavior. Ernie can take care of most of his custodial needs most days; occasionally, he will exhibit a higher level of need: he will become disoriented and lose his ability to remember what he is doing, where he is, and who people around him are. Ernie also wakes up during the night and goes outside looking to see if there is anybody out there calling his name or knocking on his door, probably due to audio hallucinations that he later forgets experiencing.

Ernie's niece made arrangements with a home care agency to provide services for Ernie that included twenty-four-hour care with an in-home non-medical health aide. This level of care included coverage from several different health aides to make seamless coverage. Ernie met this arrangement with significant resistance because he felt this represented the loss of his independence. He would argue with his health aides, accuse them of stealing from him, and refuse to eat meals they prepared for him. The agency continued to send several different aides, but Ernie would not agree to let any of them come back and would find one reason or another for their dismissal.

Finally, Ernie and his niece discussed this matter together and decided to compromise. Ernie was uncomfortable having a stranger in his home while he was sleeping, while his niece was uncomfortable with the idea of having Ernie alone all day and night. The compromise they reached included a shorter shift for health aides: someone would be there only during the daytime and early evening while Ernie was awake, not only to keep him company, but also to shop for groceries with him, prepare meals for him, and eat with him.

With this arrangement, and with Ernie now feeling he had some control over the decisions that affected his life so dramatically, he did in fact accept the next health aide the agency sent to his home. She came to his home most days of the week and stayed most of the day, taking care of the house and the meals by shopping, cleaning, and doing laundry; taking care of the bills and banking; preparing meals and eating with Ernie; providing transportation to and from medical appointments; and providing companionship for Ernie.

Ernie's symptoms progressed rapidly and so did his level of need. Ernie's niece arranged with the agency for a team of health aides to provide more and more care until eventually he was receiving twenty-four-hour coverage. But by this point, was willing to accept this arrangement. He had already established a rapport with his first health aid and this friendship served as a kind of bridge to the others. He knew what to expect and had had a good experience so far.

Assisted-Living Facilities

Assisted living can be a good residential option for people suffering from dementia who want or need help with some of the activities of daily living. Assisted-living facilities provide residents with help doing things like cooking meals, getting to and from the bathroom in the middle of the night, housekeeping chores, and traveling to outside errands.

If your loved one needs more personal care than you are able to provide them at home (either with or without the help of others), then an assisted-living facility may be an appropriate choice for you and your loved one. Your loved one may thrive in the community of assisted living, where independence is encouraged while twenty-four-hour supervision is available.

Residents are encouraged to do what they can for themselves: personalized plans are developed to accommodate an individual's needs while celebrating his strengths. Generally, assisted living is a residential-type living facility, ranging from individual or roommate-style apartments to renovated motels; some require shared room living while others provide private living quarters. They also can provide private kitchens or common dining rooms. Most facilities have some social and recreational activities for the residents.

Services Provided by Most Assisted-Living Facilities

- Meals, snacks, beverages
- Assistance with activities of daily living including: eating, bathing, dressing, going to the bathroom, and walking
- Housekeeping and room cleaning services
- Transportation
- Medical and health providers' services
- Security services
- Resident's personal security
- Exercise and diet (with dietician consultation or supervision)
- Medication management
- Laundry services
- Social and recreational activities
- Twenty-four-hour staff availability

How to Choose an Assisted-Living Facility

Assisted-living facilities differ considerably from one another, so you should take your time when choosing an assisted-living facility for your loved one. This variety can cause this task to feel overwhelming; however, the positive side is that you have a good chance of finding a facility that will be a good fit for both you and your loved one.

Try not to get overwhelmed as you begin your search for the perfect facility. Place a higher value on how you feel about the residents and staff than the specific amenities. You can always augment your loved one's physical space and personal services, but her experience with the people around her is going to mean a lot. Look for a facility with an engaging social environment, with friendly residents and caring and knowledgeable staff. Make sure that you feel the facility is a place where your loved one will fit in and develop new meaningful relationships because this is what will determine the quality of her day-to-day living experience.

What to Consider in Staff

They should have plenty of time for the residents without feeling rushed or hurried

They should appear interested in the residents and their needs

They should interact with the residents with warmth and care

They should handle emergencies competently

What to Consider in the Residents

They should appear happy and content

They should seem to enjoy interacting with one another

They should seem like people whom your loved one would enjoy getting to know and spending their time with

There should be hobbies or groups on site that look interesting to you and your loved one

Practical Considerations When Choosing an Assisted-Living Facility

The facility you select for your loved one should feel like a friendly place that is safe and comfortable—like a place that you would enjoy being. Don't place too high a value on how fancy the furniture is or whether the food is of the gourmet variety, but rather consider how comfortable your loved one will be with the people living in the facility and how friendly and caring the staff are.

What feels homey to one person might not feel at all homey to someone else. Some people prefer something small and cozy, while others would prefer something outdoorsy and with a garden and animals. Be sure to consider your loved one's preferences when choosing the facility.

Every facility offers a variety of social activities for their residents. Explore these options to find a facility that offers activities that match your loved one's interests. Some facilities have gymnasiums or access to one; other facilities have access to a library or chapel, while others still have access to activities off-site and provide transportation to places like swimming pools and shopping centers.

There's an enormous variety in the types of food different facilities can serve. You should choose a facility that serves food your loved one likes. Some facilities serve different foods, and the residents can choose what they would like to eat. The food should be well prepared and nutritious and appetizing.

When health issues arise, there should be protocols in place, and the residents should be made aware of them well in advance of any emergency. Explore the policies about how high a level of care the facility will be able to provide should your loved one develop a more serious medical condition. Would your loved one need to be transferred to a facility with more medical care available if he developed a higher level of need, or would they be able to stay at this facility to be taken care of?

There are state and local licensing requirements that the facility should be in compliance with. Check with your own state to understand what the standards are for your area, because they differ from state to state. You can also check with the Better Business Bureau to see if any complaints have been lodged against the facility.

The Move to Assisted Living

This can be a very stressful event even under the best of circumstances. Some ways you can support your loved one during this move are discussed below.

The loss of independence that accompanies the move from home into assisted living might be overwhelming, but acknowledging your loved one's feelings of loss can be helpful to her grief process. Even when your loved one willingly chooses to move to assisted living, grief and feelings of loss are a natural consequence of this move. Leaving one's home is a huge transition. Don't minimize her feelings or focus excessively on the other aspects of the move. Use empathy and sympathy to validate her feelings of loss and give her time to adjust to the new situation.

Telephones and visits can be tremendously helpful to your loved one while he is adjusting to his new environment. Family members' reassurance that he is still loved and cared for can be helpful. Whenever possible, continue to include your loved one in family events like birthdays, weekend rituals (such as seeing a movie, shopping, or going to church), and holiday celebrations. Remembering your loved one with cards and gifts sent through the mail makes them feel special when they live far away.

It is natural to expect your loved one to have worries and feel frightened about moving to a new environment; process these concerns together. Try not to assume that all complaints are just part of your loved one's situation. Expect there will be a challenging period of adjustment for your loved one, with real challenges for her. Taking her concerns seriously and taking some time talking with her about her worries will help her adjust to her new environment. Working through these challenges with you will help your loved one feel more confident in her new environment and better able to navigate future challenges independently.

A personalized living space in her new environment will help your loved one feel at home more quickly. Your loved one will feel more at home with their own belongings around them. Take some time to visit your loved one's new home so you can help her decorate. And make it homier. But be careful not to make it your rendition of homey, because it is their home.

Planning and Paying for an Assisted-Living Facility

The majority of costs for assisted-living facilities will probably be self-paid because most health insurance policies do not cover these costs. Cost will therefore be a consideration when evaluating assisted living for your loved one. You will find assisted-living facilities that are operated by both for-profit and nonprofit organizations and can cost from approximately upward of $10,000 a month or more, depending on where you live. For many people, this can be a major investment, so take some time to develop a budget and prioritize your needs.

While evaluating an assisted-living facility, the cost is not always positively correlated with the value. Examine what the facility has regarding your needs, the quality and responsiveness of the staff, and how friendly the residents as a community feel to you and your loved one.

The billing procedure of the facility is also something you should consider. Some facilities use a flat fee and charge add-on costs for additional services. An example of this type of billing would be when a resident begins to require a higher level of care, and the facility would begin to charge a higher fee for this as an add-on service. It is good business to discuss fees before you sign a contract. If a facility is vague with you regarding their fees, do not use this facility. It is your right to have access to this information. If a facility is not willing to provide you with this information, find another facility.

Ask about past rate increases. You don't want to encounter unexpected sharp rate increases in the future. Naturally, you can't predict the future, but you can ask about how rates have been increased in the past.

Assisted living provides a higher level of care than independent living while providing a lower level of care than skilled nursing facilities. Assisted living or in-home care might be an appropriate choice for individuals who require only minimal assistance. If your loved is beginning to develop a high level of medical needs, you may need to consider skilled-nursing facilities or other facilities with skilled medical care.

Skilled-Nursing Facilities

A skilled-nursing facility provides a higher level of care than assisted living while providing a lower level of care than a hospital. Assistance with getting in and out of bed, eating and meal preparation, bathing and dressing, and laundry and housekeeping is provided at skilled-nursing facilities. However, skilled-nursing facilities differ from other senior housing facilities in that they also provide a higher level of medical care than is possible in other housing. Medical professionals provide patients with medical care, and a nurse or other medical professional is almost always available should the need for their services arise.

The environment and decor varies among skilled-nursing facilities. For example, some facilities offer single rooms, while in other facilities, only shared rooms are available. Some rooms may

have their own kitchenettes, others may share a community dining atmosphere, and still others may provide meals in the room.

Not all skilled-nursing facilities are currently using the medical model for their layout, although this was once the case. Some
skilled-nursing facilities have transitions into the more modern
model of patient care, where the patient is the focus of care. These
communities are smaller, with patient-strength-based features
like independent cooking facilities and a higher staff-per-patient
ratio.

When to Consider a Skilled-Nursing Facility

The decision to move a loved one into a skilled-nursing facility is never easy, and with it comes feelings of guilt, shame, and
anger. The decision to move may be sudden, or it may have been
a long and well-thought-out decision, but there are going to be
difficulties for both you and your loved one with this decision.

If your loved one is considering a move to this level of care,
he's probably already receiving a significant amount of care and
has therefore already been assessed. If not, a thorough medical
and psychological assessment is necessary, so evaluate his needs
and strengths so you can make a well-informed decision about
the level of care he needs and how to best provide this.

Consider your loved one's needs and where and how they will
best be met. If you cannot safely provide the level of care needed
in your own home, then can the care be augmented with in-home
services or help from family or community resources? If this is
still not enough to fill in the gaps, then moving to assisted living
or a skilled-nursing facility may be the best fit for your loved one.

Consider the fit of your loved one's needs and the availability of the primary caregiver. Caregivers often have many other

demands on their time like work, other personal needs, and their own health. It's not possible for one person to provide twenty- four hour care alone and caregiving is a twenty-four hour a day job. It is sometimes possible for others to provide assistance in care giving duties but this is not always the case. Other times respite and adult day care programs may be helpful. Eventually, it may be wise to consider whether home care service are too expensive or if the need is too great to provide quality care for your loved one.

Consider the length of time your loved one will need this level of care. Will they need to be in a skilled-nursing facility permanently, or will their stay more likely be on a temporary basis? Consider temporary options from family members, community resources, or additional in-home services. However, if your loved one might likely need a longer term of care, these options might be expensive or inconvenient.

Finding the Right Skilled-Nursing Facility

Medical and custodial care is provided in skilled-nursing facilities; this is some of the highest level of care a facility provides. Your loved one may not require this level of care at this time. If you're not sure that you or your loved one needs this level of care at this time or for the long term, you may wish to explore other types of senior housing, like home care, to identify what will best fit your loved one's needs.

It can be a daunting task to find a skilled-nursing facility for your loved one, especially when you are under the additional pressure of worrying about their increasing health concerns. Here are some things to consider while thinking about your options:

Start with referrals. Ask your family physician or specialist for any recommendations they may have. Or you may know friends or family members who have used different facilities. Knowing someone with firsthand experience with a facility can help you make well-informed choices. However, remember your loved one's needs may differ from others'.

When evaluating a skilled-nursing facility, consider whether it is a good match for your loved one's needs. Every facility has a different area of expertise so try to find one that specializes in what your loved one needs.

Another consideration is how far the facility is from your home. In general, the more convenient the facility is to get to, the easier it is for family and friends to visit.

Now that you have some facilities to consider, you will need to make some in-person visits to evaluate them further. There is only so much you can learn about your choices by telephone or online; it's what you see in person that will help you make your final choice. Once you arrive on-site, you will be evaluating not only the facility itself, but the residents and the staff as well.

What to look for in staff and residents

The facility you choose should be well-staffed round-the-clock seven days per week. Ask about staff retention and the length of time staff has been there. Think about how engaging the staff are with you and how much time they are willing to spend with you, because this is probably how they will treat your loved one when you are not there. Are the staff well trained regarding the health needs of your loved one? Consider how individual health needs are taken care of. Evaluate policies for injuries and if there is adequate staffing in case of emergencies.

Consider how the residents seem to look and feel in their living environment. Do they look engaged or do they seem depressed, isolated, and over-medicated? Look for happy, active residents who look like people your loved one would have something in common with and get along well with. Consider how other residents respond to you: are they apathic or are they engaging? If you can obtain permission, stay for a community meal to see how the food is served and how the residents enjoy the food. Evaluate how much assistance residents are receiving with meals and how much independence they are encouraged to retain. If you have an opportunity, ask other family members how their loved one has felt about living in this facility.

What to look for in the facility itself

Examine the facility for its cleanliness and odors that cannot be explained. Are there strong odors or scents of deodorizers covering up the smell of urine? Evaluate the meal-preparation area and the food being served. This should be clean and appealing, and the food should look nutritious.

Consider the feel and ambiance for a homely feeling. Does the area seem sterile or medical, or do you see decorations and personal belongings around that look like they belong to the residents? How large is the community? If the community is too large, your loved one may feel as though she's lost in the crowd rather than feel at home.

Consider the social environment and what types of activities are available for the residents. If activities are offered that are off the premises, does the facility offer transportation? Are the residents interested in the activities that are offered?

Think about the quality of care provided at the facility. For example, if your loved one has Alzheimer's, is this facility capable of taking care of patients with this condition? Are they properly staffed for this—do they have knowledge of the medical and behavioral needs for patients with this condition? Ask how many patients they currently have with this condition and how many patients they have accommodated in the past with this condition.

Understanding Skilled-Nursing Facility Costs

Skilled-nursing facilities can be expensive, and depending on the state you live in, costs can vary widely. There are strict and complicated limitations of insurance in coverage of costs: For example, Medicare covers only limited stays in skilled-nursing facilities. Custodial care is not covered by Medicare if that is the only care needed (citation needed).

If your loved one's income and assets are limited, Medicaid might be an option. However, each facility has different regulations regarding acceptance of Medicaid. There are types of insurance you can purchase that might cover these types of costs in the future. If you suspect that your loved one may need extended nursing home care in the future, check the provisions of his plan to see what portion of skilled nursing facility coverage is covered.

The Moving Process

Adjusting to life transitions takes time for the entire family. Allow everyone time to adjust to their own feelings and work through how they are feeling, and expect to feel confused and conflicted at times. Trying to deny your anger and grief or refusing to acknowledge the difficulties of the transition will only intensify these feelings.

Whenever possible, encourage your loved one to participate in making the decisions about which skilled-nursing facility is best for them. Encourage your loved one to come with you to visit and assess the facilities and have a meaningful role in the decision-making process. If it isn't possible for your loved one to visit facilities with you, then try to consider his preferences while you are evaluating facilities. Take photos for him to examine and bring home pamphlets and advertising materials. If your loved one is in a facility that is not near your home, you can still stay close in touch with telephone calls, e-mails, and cards. Continue to invite your loved one to family traditions and holiday celebrations after they have moved to their new facility.

Choosing a Hospital

It can be overwhelming and confusing to find the best quality hospital for the care you need. Quality should be your first consideration when choosing a hospital because research shows that some hospitals that regularly do a greater number of a specific type of procedure, have a better quality outcome and a higher patient satisfaction rating.

The Joint Commission

The Joint Commission, formerly the Joint Commission on Accreditation of Healthcare Organizations, is an organization that accredits health-care facilities. Look for a hospital that has approval from the Joint Commission and is rated highly by other state or consumer or other groups. Find a hospital where your doctor has privileges, if that is important to you. Find one that is covered by your health plan, has experience with your loved one's condition, has had success with that condition, and checks on itself and works to improve its own quality of care.

Hospitals typically choose on their own be analyzed by the Joint Commission to determine if they meet certain quality standards. The standards address the specific quality of staffing and equipment used in the hospital and the hospital's success record in treating and curing patients. If the Joint Commission determines that a hospital meets those standards, they accredit it. The hospital participates in quarterly reviews. Most hospitals participate in this program, and participation is voluntary.

The Joint Commission develops a report on each hospital that it surveys. The report lists accreditation status, reporting how the hospital preformed on each of six levels of analysis. This report includes critical evaluation of each area looked at with any need for a revisit or if accreditation was received without conditions. The report for each hospital is also reviewed with national results as comparison data.

The Joint Commission's performance reports are available on all hospitals they review by calling 630-792-5800; or check its Web site at www.jointcommission.org for any hospital's performance report or for its accreditation status.

Local Consumer Groups

Consider collecting data from local consumer groups. This process of checks and balances encourages hospitals to improve their quality of care, as well as providing vital information for consumers. Checks and balances is a excellent reason to look for and use consumer information about hospitals. You can obtain data about hospital performance in your area by contacting your state department of health, health-care council, or hospital association. Your doctor will probably have valuable opinions regarding quality of care for the hospital you are considering

By Specialty

You may also choose a hospital by its specialty. For example, "general" hospitals handle a wide range of routine conditions, while specialty hospitals have a lot of experience with certain conditions or certain groups: for example, you may be able to choose a general hospital for gallbladder surgery, a specialty hospital if you need care for a heart condition, and a specialty hospital for your children.

When choosing your health plan, be mindful of which hospitals your coverage will allow you to use and where your physician has credentials, because this is probably where you will be receiving services.

Once a physician or hospital has successfully completed many of a certain procedure, they will become more proficient with their skills. Consider this when choosing a hospital, and choose one that has expertise with your needs. Evaluate your hospital's statistics regarding:

How many procedures similar to the one you will need have been performed at this hospital?

How many times has your physician performed the procedure you will need and how successful has he been with his procedures?

Evaluate the hospital's patient outcomes not only regarding your condition but in all areas in the hospital.

Outcome Studies

Outcome studies are reports published by some health departments regarding patient outcomes on certain procedures. These studies show, for example, how well patients do after having a certain procedure like bypass surgery. Such studies can help you compare which hospitals and surgeons have had the most success with a given procedure.

Keeping a record of patient outcomes is how hospitals improve their quality of care not only for individual procedures but also as an organization as a whole. Quality of care is becoming increasingly important to hospitals. There are several ways to track patient outcomes. For example, tracking patient injuries and infections for specific procedures or tracking general patient outcomes for specific procedures are methods that can produce data that can be tracked and compared to other hospital's outcome data.

Speak with the hospital quality management department about how it handles patient quality of care. Also, ask if you may see any data from recent patient satisfaction surveys. These will tell you how other patients have rated the quality of their care

It can be overwhelming to think about the many options available when considering a move to a higher level of care for your loved one. Take your time, consider all your options and make a well informed decision.

9. Hospice and Palliative Care

Hospice care and Palliative care are a range of treatments available for end-of-life care that not nearly enough patients and physicians are fully aware of. This section provides a general discussion about Hospice and Palliative care but it is recommended that you contact a professional who specializes in this area when your loved one is ready for this range of treatment.

Hospice Care

In order for a patient to become eligible for hospice benefits, they must meet a specific set of criteria established by Medicare. Medicare regulations are most often the standard used because Medicare pays for a large portion of hospice benefits. Of these criteria, often the most challenging for a patient with dementia to meet is the consideration that they have no more than six months to live. For a patient with dementia, this can be very difficult to determine. Within these standards set forth by Medicare, the main focus is on physical deterioration; to be eligible for hospice care, a patient must be:

- unable to walk unassisted
- unable to dress him- or herself
- unable to bathe or see to grooming needs without help
- unable to control bowel and bladder
- unable to converse effectively (though some language may remain)

The patient must have at least one additional serious medical issue. For example, evidence of profound nutritional problems, severe bedsores, or kidney problems.

When a hospice patient with dementia exceeds the six-month limit, it is possible to be recertified for successive thirty-day periods in order to continue receiving Medicare coverage. Dementia can be a slowly progressing disease and it is therefore difficult to determine when end of life is near. Hospice can be an option for individuals with dementia-related disorders during end-stage, even though end-stage is difficult to define. Therefore, patients with dementia-related disorders can face difficulties meeting hospice eligibilities requirements.

Hospice services are a group of services, and it might seem that some of the services might be unlikely to benefit people with dementia. For example, because people with dementia are so severely impaired cognitively, they cannot make use of psychotherapy because they have lost their ability to communicate with language.

However, there are many other hospice services that might impact the patient in positive ways. For example, pet therapy—holding and petting a small, gentle animal—as well as music therapy can have many nurturing outcomes for people with dementia. These techniques do not require that the patient have language capabilities to benefit from the intervention and to enjoy the time spent doing the activity.

It is believed that people with severe dementia may also derive comfort from friendly voices when being read to, even without understanding what is being said. The benefit is still gained whether or not the patient recognizes the reader; what is important for the benefit to be received is that the voice they hear is calm and soothing.

Support for Caregivers

Depending on many factors, prognosis for someone with dementia can range from eight to twenty years. Providing care for a loved one with dementia can be exhausting and draining in many ways: physically, emotionally, and financially. Often, this responsibility can far exceed what any family member can provide. Hospice can augment the efforts of family members and help loved ones remain in their homes for as long as possible. The family works as a team to provide the basic daily care while the hospice team complements these efforts with the skilled work of social workers, nurses, and community volunteers. Some hospice programs also provide respite care to give caregivers a break from their caregiving responsibilities.

Many hospice arrangements are available. As your loved one progresses to late-stage dementia, the increasing needs of more severe symptoms and a higher level of needs might convince your family to seek a higher level of care. Several different hospice arrangements remain available at every level of care, including residential care hospice and hospice care provided at a care facility.

Finally, hospice offers bereavement counseling for the family members and close friends who are affected by the death of their loved one. There are many different ways this part of the hospice process can be carried out. Each person will grieve differently.

Eligibility and Financing

Many hospice programs are covered by Medicare while many are not; this is important to find out while researching your hospice program. Speak to others who have used the program you are interested in, or research programs that a friend or relative refers you to. Use a program that's conveniently located, and check them out with your local Chamber of Commerce and Better Business Bureau.

Palliative Care

Palliative care is something patients with dementia can benefit from because they are often unable to express their pain; the focus of palliative care is providing comfort while not necessarily providing a cure. Palliative care can be part of hospice care services, but it can also be a service when a patient is not dying. Palliative care focuses on providing comfort for the patient, but this might be a benefit for patients who are not dying as well as for patients while they approach death. There are the several differences that distinguish palliative care from hospice care.

Pain management is the goal of palliative care; the patient does not have to have hospice status to receive palliative care. The patient may be undergoing a curative treatment while receiving palliative care and in fact recover, at which point palliative care would no longer be necessary. This differs from the goal of hospice treatment because the hospice patient will not seek a curative treatment and will not recover and will have less than six months to live.

Palliative care is also referred to as comfort care; it provides comfort by relieving distress while the patient moves either toward wellness or toward death. Palliative care looks at dying as part of the normal human condition and supports this process with dignity and respect for the patient's wishes.

Both palliative care and hospice care are regularly offered in hospitals, nursing homes, and assisted-living facilities. Although such services are available in the home, they're not necessarily provided only in the home, for example, hospice care and palliative care can be provided at any level of care facility.

Hospice care is a regularly approved program for payments by Medicare, Medicaid, or other insurance carriers. However, palliative care is not always regularly approved by all insurance programs and is therefore a benefit that must be evaluated by a patient's individual insurance provider.

When Is Palliative Care Needed?

Palliative care is considered at the discretion of the patient and the attending physician. Usually someone from the hospice team like the physician, the patient, or the patient's family can request a palliative care consult. Currently, there are no standardized guidelines (as is the case with hospice care) for when palliative care is indicated.

Palliative care includes a team of a physician, a nurse, a social worker, someone who coordinates care for the family, and may also include a chaplain. The care may discontinue once the patient is discharged from the inpatient facility, or it could continue after the patient returns home. The palliative care team—especially the nurse , social worker, and chaplain—will meet with the patient and the family to explore the loved one's physical symptoms; the family's social, emotional, spiritual, and financial needs; their personal priorities; and the losses they are experiencing. The team also will consult with the primary-care physician regarding his or her concerns and needs. The team will subsequently make recommendations for care and connect the patient to possible community resources. The palliative care team will also provide palliative care consults to nursing homes, the patients, and their families if there are uncontrolled symptoms or unmet needs.

Benefits of Palliative Care

Palliative care is a relatively new field and its benefits of are numerous. Filling a potential gap between standard medical care and hospice care, palliative care offers personalized care for patients at many different stages of illness. Some patients may not be prepared to accept the limitations of aggressive treatments associated with their illness and the concurrent symptoms of such treatments, while others may be in transition from curative treatment to longer-term care and symptom management. Still other patients may be seeking a more proactive approach to the management of pain and symptoms at each stage of treatment.

Health-care professionals and families also benefit from a team approach and the support delivered in an atmosphere of concern for quality of life and the well-being of the patient beyond the physical aspect alone. Symptom management, spiritual care, and concern for the welfare of those impacted by serious illness are hallmarks of palliative care. Studies have shown that involvement in palliative care often leads to not only improved quality of life for both the patient and the caregiver but also to an extended life expectancy. Palliative care also helps to lower patient financial cost and stress.

10. Decisions about Late-Stage Care

Late-stage care is characterized by several significant changes from other stages of care; however, there is no definitive moment when this happens. Some areas of care may gradually shift and no longer be curative, while other areas may still be curative. This can be a confusing time for caregivers and family members. The focus of care eventually shifts from curative measures to palliative care and comfort measures. End-of-life care is more than caregiving choices, and the family members begin the part of the grieving process that moves them toward acceptance. Your loved one's final days can be a time of reconnecting for both of you.

As your loved one's illness progresses, it will become evident that he needs more care than you can provide in order for them to proceed with comfort and dignity. In the final stages of a life-limiting illness, with increased attention and assistance at a higher level of care, your loved one can continue to live in the familiar surroundings of their own home, or you may wish to transition them to a facility that can provide a high level of care. Depending on the nature of the dementia and comorbid illness, and the patient's circumstances, this late-stage period may last a matter of days, weeks, or months.

End-stage care can be overwhelming even for professional health-care providers. Feeling lost is normal. You might feel numb or confused when faced with decisions about care for your loved one; it's okay to ask other family members to help you at this time. Decide on care decisions as a group, and use advance care directives and power of attorney that you have prepared in advance with your loved one. Rely on the assistance of your hospice care team, community resources, and spiritual community.

You and your care team will determine when end-stage care begins. There are no guidelines for exactly when this will occur, just as there are no exact guidelines regarding what this type of care will look like. Develop this plan tailored to your loved one's needs under your care team's direction.

When thinking about end-stage care, consider how many times your loved one has visited the hospital's emergency room within the last year for similar issues. Has your loved one been treated many times for similar conditions without improving their quality of life, or has their condition progressively declined? Does your loved one refuse to go to the hospital for conditions that require medical attention, or do they wish to remain at home to receive care? Has your loved one been admitted to a hospital for symptoms of different conditions with an overall decline in their general medical health? Have they stopped authorizing medical treatment, or are they hiding symptoms from family members?

End-Stage Symptoms

Symptoms in the final stages of life will vary from patient to patient and from illness to illness, but some symptoms are universal and can be expected to be seen in all patients. Use caution when identifying these symptoms because they can also be symptoms of other stages of some illnesses and are not always an indication that death is near.

Cooling of the skin

Your loved one's extremities will begin to feel cool when you touch them, and you may notice some color change as well. This is due to a normal decrease in the circulation of blood to these areas because the body reserves blood for vital organs and the body's ability to produce circulation is limited. Cover your loved one with a blanket to keep them warm.

Increased Sleeping

Your loved one may begin to need more sleep and rest and might seem to have difficulty communicating with their environment. At times, they may seem difficult to wake. This is due to a metabolic decrease, and at this time your loved one will need you to hold their hand or touch them to rouse them before communicating, or they may not be aware you are trying to communicate with them. Use a calm and gentle voice when speaking with your loved one; no need to speak loudly, because this will likely distress them. Try to spend more time with your loved one while they are awake, and allow them to continue sleeping when they are naturally resting. Remember that although your loved one may look like they are sleeping, they might still be able to hear you, so be mindful of what you say while in their room where they can hear you. Hearing is usually the last sense that a person loses.

Disorientation/ Confusion

Expect confusion regarding people, time, and where they are as well as who you are and what is happening. Try not to make your loved one guess, but rather just identify yourself before you speak or identify a situation as a reference to what you are going to tell them. Speak in simple, short sentences and be truthful about the information you convey.

Incontinence

Your loved one will begin to lose control of bowel and bladder muscles, resulting in incontinence. Focus on cleanliness and comfort for your loved one, and consult your hospice team for the best way to accomplish this task.

Congestion

Your loved one will begin to experience a non-painful, deep-rolling sound emanating from her chest. The sound resembles that of a phlegm-producing cough, and this can get to be a very loud sound. This is a normal experience and is the result of decreased fluid consumption, which causes the impairment in the ability to cough productively. Turn your loved one's head to the side and allow the secretions to flow out naturally. Use a warm, moist washcloth to keep the face clean. This is a noisy experience; however, the noise is not positively correlated with pain.

Restlessness

Your loved one might appear restless and pull at the bed-sheets, call out, or pull at his night clothing. A decrease in the oxygen supply to cortical structures resulting in metabolic changes causes these behaviors. Allow your loved one to continue with these behaviors, and don't attempt to restrain them. Speak calmly while providing a gentle massage and use soft, soothing music.

Decrease in Urine Production

Expect a decrease in your loved one's urine as well as a darkening in color. With the decrease in fluid consumption and decrease in circulation, the darkened urine color and decrease in urine production is normal. Your hospice nurse will make an evaluation to see if a catheter is necessary.

Fluid and Food Intake Decrease

Your loved one may experience a decrease in appetite and thirst, making use of little or no food or fluid. The body will not be using energy for digestion, but rather, it will be using its energy only on vital tasks like respiration and circulation. If your loved one refuses food, accept their need not to eat, and allow them to rest or sleep. Offer them slivers of ice or flavored ice or juice. If your loved one is no longer able to swallow, you may use a syringe to administer fluids into their mouth. You might use a cool moistened washcloth placed on their forehead to comfort them.

Breathing Pattern Change

Your loved one may begin to breathe irregularly. Several patterns exist: one pattern consists of breathing irregularly; for example, shallow breaths with periods of no breathing of five to thirty seconds and up to a full minute. Your loved one may also experience periods of rapid shallow panting. These patterns are very common and indicate decrease in circulation in the internal organs. When you notice irregular breathing in your loved one, try elevating his head or turning them on their side for comfort.

Withdrawal

Your loved one might have a withdrawn or coma-like appearance. This is because they are preparing to let go and is moving away from relationships and their environment. Continue speaking to your loved one with your normal voice, say your goodbyes, and let them know whatever you need them to know. This will help your loved one to let go.

Vision-like experiences

Your loved one may be experiencing hallucinations that are very real to them at this time. Do not try to convince them that this is not happening to try to explain it away. Honor their experience and try to hold it in a beautiful light for them. Their hallucinating is an indication that they are letting go of his environment and this life and preparing for death in a way that will not frighten them. Try to honor and affirm this experience and know this is a normal reaction to death.

Talking, sitting, walking, eating, or making sense of the world may be difficult or impossible for your loved one during late-stage care. Routine activities—including bathing, feeding, toileting, dressing, and turning—may require total support and increased physical strength on the part of the caregiver. This is when a higher level of care is necessary because support by professional assistants, a hospice team, or nursing services is the only way to manage your loved one's care.

When demands become overwhelming, respite care can provide you and other caregivers a break from the intensity of providing round-the-clock care. Hospice volunteers may relieve caregivers and spend time with patients for short periods of time for your much needed self-care, or a hospice facility can accommodate the patient for inpatient stays for longer periods of time while caregivers take longer breaks.

Knowing a loss is eminent can result in feelings of numbness, anxiety, and sadness. Bereavement specialists and spiritual advisors can be supportive and helpful during this time by assisting with final preparation as well as spiritual support.

Getting Ready for End-of-Life Needs

Being clear with your loved one about end-of-life wishes provides family members with clearly understood directions regarding the patient's preferences about treatment for end-of-life care. Family members can be free to use their time and energy for their own grief process rather than worry about their loved one's wishes. Conversations regarding things like medical treatment, end-of-life wishes, and placement should be held as soon as possible. Consideration should be given to things like hospice and palliative care services, spiritual needs, and memorial and cultural preferences before they are needed, so when it is time, they will be in place.

As discussed in chapter four, financial and legal advice should be considered early while your loved one can participate. Legal documents such as a power of attorney and an advanced directive can explain a patient's wishes so there will be no confusion among family members in the future.

If there is no living will or advance directive for your loved one, act on what you know or feel their wishes are as you determine by their values. Consider past conversations and events from when their values were salient and determine what the person would like to do with their end-of-life care from this vantage point.

As your loved one's illness progresses, be prepared to experience increased stress yourself and between family members. The painful feelings of fear, guilt, and loss can cause conflict and remorse between family members, and this is normal. Don't let this get in the way of the decisions you need to make regarding your loved one's medical care and final arrangements. Get help from bereavement counselors or a private therapist if necessary.

Have someone within your family who will serve as the primary decision maker and manage information. Let one person serve as a coordinator of your loved one's wishes and be the main support person. Implementing end-of-life wishes takes communication, and it is not something everyone is able to do.

Including children, when possible, can be nurturing. Provide your children with honest, age-appropriate information about your family member's condition and any changes they perceive in you. Children can be profoundly affected by situations they don't understand, and may come to inaccurate conclusions without appropriate information. Children may benefit from drawing pictures or using puppets to express feelings, and hearing stories that explain events in terms they can easily understand.

End-Stage Care and Placement Options

With the progression of the illnesses comorbid to dementia, your loved one will need a higher level of care than you might be able to provide at home by yourself or with the help of other family members or friends or even with the assistance of in-home services or community resources. This is the time to consider getting additional in-home help or for your loved one to be moved into a hospice or other care facility. Often, it is possible to help your loved one to remain in the comfort of their own home during the final stages of life, in familiar surroundings with family and loved ones nearby.

End-stage dementia presents difficulty with multiple changes in the patient's environment. If you are planning to move your loved one to a care facility, it's better to move him before he reaches the end-stage of his illness.

Hospice is an option for patients whose life expectancy is six months or less, and can be provided in the patient's home or in a care facility. Hospice services can include palliative care, which is pain and symptom relief to provide your loved with the highest quality of life possible during their final days. Once pain is removed from the picture, the hope is that you and your loved one will be able to focus on what is important to you during the time that is remaining.

Family members are actively involved in the treatment when hospice care is provided at home, while supervised by a team of professional health care providers. The hospice care team is available to the patient twenty-four hours a day and makes regular visits to provide care like therapy and bathing and assessments. The hospice team provides emotional and spiritual support as directed by the patient. The team also provides support to the family. When deciding if you can take care of your loved one at home, you should consider the following questions:

Has your loved one made their wishes clear regarding end-of-life care that include continuing to receive care at home?

Are you or another family member able to provide qualified, dependable support for your loved one twenty-four hours a day?

Is your loved one's home, or your home, able to accommodate the special medical equipment necessary to provide proper care?

If your loved one is able to make use of transportation, are you able to provide this? Can you provide transportation for your loved one in case of emergencies?

Do you have access to medical professionals for your loved one's non-emergency needs?

Do you have the physical strength and knowledge necessary to lift and move and turn your loved one?

Will you be able to provide twenty-four-hour care for your loved one and still maintain your own responsibilities?

How will you cope with the emotional challenges of providing twenty-four- hour care of your loved one?

Providing Emotional Comfort

Emotional needs during the end-of-life stage differ from patient to patient. However, some universal experiences include worry about loss of control and dignity as physical abilities decline. Becoming a burden to loved ones is also common experience as is a fear of being abandoned. Emotional comfort can be provided to patients simply by keeping the patient company.

Process your own painful feelings of grief with someone else, not your loved one. Spend time holding your loved one's hand, reading to them, talking to them, or watching a movie together. Allow the patient to express fears of death. Try to listen to your loved one as they talk about their fears of death and how they are accepting what is happening to them. It can be painful to hear a loved one talk about leaving family and friends behind, but talking about their fears can help them com to terms with what's happening. Just offer them empathy and listen to them without trying to 'fix' anything.

Encouraging your loved one to place their life in review is a good way for them to make sense of their life's events. Help them celebrate what they did well and witness their life in a "life review." Allow them to reminisce their precious memories. Celebrate your loved one's joys and offer a rephrase for what they do not feel proud of. For example, you might say "Imagine that! You worked at the same place for forty years, what reliable employee and good friend you must have been to your colleagues."

Reassure your loved one that you understand and will honor their wishes—such as advance directives and durable power of attorney—and you will carry them out even if you don't agree with them. Be open and honest about all information regarding the health care and personal care of your loved one. Be communicative and up front about everything concerning your loved one. Understand her need for privacy and respect her concerns.

The period during which your loved one is "dying," when body systems are shutting down and death is imminent, can last from days to weeks. For some patients this is a peaceful experience, while for others this seems to be a fight against the inevitable. Try to reassure your loved one that you are here and it is okay to let go and die. Any decisions at this time about end-of-life care must be consistent with your loved one's directives.

Assisted Suicide and Euthanasia

When the topic of assisted suicide and euthanasia comes up, many different feelings can begin to surface for different people. It can be tempting to think you would know what to do if you were in another person's place. But realistically, this is not possible to ever know.

People might contemplate ending their life for many reasons, and if the outcome of their dilemma is uncertain, then a permanent solution is a risky choice. However, when the reason for suffering is because of a terminal illness, and their suffering is guaranteed to increase until the time of their death, then this might be a reason to hasten the end of life. The question becomes not if one is going to die but rather when one is going to die. The question further becomes how one will die and with what degree of suffering one will die.

Unfortunately, the natural and extremely personal act of dying is not so simple. Laws dictate how and when one can die and by what means death can occur. Suicide is the act of intentionally causing one's own death, and this is a crime. Assisted suicide is helping one to intentionally cause their own death and in all but three stated in this country, this is also a crime. Euthanasia is the act of ending someone else's life for the purpose of ending pain and suffering, which includes passive euthanasia: for example, withholding life-sustaining measures like mechanical breathing and feeding procedures—in some instances, this is legal in this country.

One who defends the right to die might argue that euthanasia and physician-assisted suicide of terminally ill people provides the right for them to end their suffering with a quick, dignified, and compassionate death. One might further argue that the right to die is protected by the same constitutional safeguards that guarantee such rights as marriage, procreation, and the refusal or termination of life-saving medical treatment (procon.org, 2010).

Those who oppose euthanasia and physician-assisted suicide might argue that doctors have a moral responsibility to keep their patients alive as reflected by the Hippocratic Oath. They might further argue there may be only a very fuzzy boundary, is any boundary at all from euthanasia to murder, and that legalizing euthanasia will unfairly target the poor and disabled and create incentives for insurance companies to terminate lives in order to save money (procon.org, 2010).

There are individual organizations and people who support assisted suicide and euthanasia for terminally ill individuals. Some of these organizations can be found locally and some can be found in other countries. They each have different ethical and medical criteria their patients must pass before they will take them on as patients but generally they help people end their lives with dignity as they choose. A list of these organizations appears in the Resources section at the end of this book.

Assisted suicide is legal in the three American states of Oregon, Washington, and Montana. However, before one can legally use assisted suicide procedures, they must undergo rigorous legal standards. For example, in Oregon, the patient must self-administer the medication their physician prescribed. They

must be able to request the medication in writing and twice verbally, and the physician must make a recorded statement that this
act is voluntary and well informed, and that the patient has less
than six months to live.

After the patient has passed away, you might need some time
to be with your loved one, to say good-bye. Some people are
comforted by prayer, talking with loved ones, or just sitting with
their loved one at this time. It is important to take all the time you
need. There are many ways to process this experience: the next
chapter discusses the grieving process in detail.

11. Coping with Grief and Loss

Being prepared for the loss of a loved one means more than simply knowing their death is imminent. When a loved one actually dies, shock, sadness, disbelief, and unexpected feelings can result. For most people, the actual death starts the normal grieving process.

What Is Grief?

When we experience a loss, we suffer normal and painful internal feelings of the experience: this is grief, while having experienced the loss is bereavement. Whenever we experience any type of loss we can suffer emotional pain. For example, losing a job or a cherished belonging is genuinely painful. However, *grief* usually refers to the loss of a loved one through death.

Grief is a common and natural human condition. Most people outlive their spouse; usually women outlive their husbands by 75 percent, with the average age of becoming a widow being fifty-six years. Nothing can, or intends to, minimize a grief experience; but rather when thinking about others who have survived their grief, these thoughts are meant to give hope.

When the grieving process lasts more than a year, it is considered complicated grief, or prolonged grief. With complicated grief, the grief reaction intensifies and affects all the sufferer's relationships and belief systems. It can manifest in an inconsolable longing for the lost loved one at the expense of anyone else participating in the sufferer's daily life.

Anticipatory grief is a constellation of feelings we experience in reaction to knowing that our loved ones are terminally ill.

This can be an important part of the grieving process because it allows us to say good-bye, to get legal affairs in order (further discussed in chapter four), and to plan funerals and other important rituals.

What Is Mourning?

While grief is the internal experience of a loss of a loved one, mourning is the outward expression of that loss. Culturally laden rituals are usually a large part of the mourning experience that help the community in the period immediately after the loss of a loved one by providing structure. While the internal pain of grief is a more universal experience, how people mourn and express their feelings of grief is influenced by their personal, familial, cultural, religious, and societal beliefs and customs.

The entire experience of mourning is personal—from how families communicate their loved one's death and record the event for future generations, to how they understand and react to the passing, to the practices for preserving memories of their loved one. The funeral or memorial, burial, cremation, and other ways of handling the remains of the deceased are influenced by both internal and external (cultural) factors.

Formal mourning periods vary depending on cultural factors and personal preferences. Employers usually have predetermined bereavement period they allow employees. The length of time for a formal mourning period (or the amount of bereavement leave) that employers allow is determined by a combination of personal, familial, cultural, religious, and societal factors. The way in which bereaved individuals may seek support, or if they seek support al all can be influenced by culture. For example, some cultures may encourage aggrieved individuals to talk about their loss with friends, family members, and coworkers; while other cultures may not. This encouragement (or lack of it) may influence whether participating in a bereavement support group or psychotherapy is acceptable.

The Grief Process

Grief is more than a single event that occurs when you cry or when you feel sad. It includes the tears you shed when you think of a loss, but it is more. This process is a way in which we let go of our loved ones and incorporate them into our memory in a healthy way.

They ways we grieve are individual, and it is important to honor our own process. Grief is painful, but when you suffer a loss, it is important to be allowed to suffer your grief and to be supported in the ways you need to be supported. The time you need to grieve will be different than others, and the intensity of your pain will vary. Grieving is painful, but it's a necessary part of having a meaningful relationship with your loved one and receiving support throughout the process is important.

It is normal for people to begin to feel better only to feel sad again. It can be a long time before the grieving process begins to subside and sometimes, it may seem as though it will go on forever. There is no answer to how long this process will last for any specific individual, but your grieving process will be affected by circumstances like:

- the kind of relationship you had with the person who died
- the circumstances of their death
- your own life experiences
- how you processed previous losses

Initially, you might experience shock or numbness when you begin to process your grief. Gradually, as you begin to think of pragmatic or everyday ways this loss will affect your life, emotions begin to make way. You may continue to experience fleeting moments of shock and numbness, but periods of anger, disbelief, denial, loneliness, and sadness will begin to appear. This fluctuating-mood state can last for a long time. Finally, you will work out terms with your loss and accept the loss of your loved one.

Again, your first experience might be a feeling of disbelief, shock, or numbness. Expect this to continue for days to weeks, maybe longer. It's okay to feel disconnected or to feel like you are just going through the motions of your day. This is normal. You might feel moments when these feelings are stronger than at other times; these moments might be brought on by reminders of your loss. You may cry a lot. You might feel irritable, or confused. At these times of distress, you may feel agitated, have difficulty concentrating, or become forgetful. You may experience physical symptoms like pain or difficulty sleeping. You may be preoccupied with thoughts or images of your loved one. This is all normal.

Facing the Loss Brings Out Painful Emotions

Eventually, as the numbness begins to dissipate and you begin to realize the effects the loss will have on your life, reality hits you. This is when you can begin to do what's called confrontation of your loss. In this stage your feelings are most intense and painful because you are no longer numb. Healing starts to take place at this time because you are coping with the meaning of your loss, and now you can start to make changes in your life.

This can be a time of significant distress, and you may seem disorganized or confused. You may experience difficulty remembering things or concentrating. You may have difficulty with daily activities like making telephone calls or shopping for groceries.

Weeks to months may go by before you pass through this stage into the final stage of grieving.

Common Symptoms of Grief

Although we all grieve differently, the following are some symptoms most common in the bereaved:

- difficulty thinking and concentrating
- restlessness
- anxiety
- fear
- changes in appetite (weight loss, weight gain)
- sadness
- dreams of the deceased (or even hallucinations or "visions" in which you briefly hear or see the deceased)
- changes in sleep patterns (sleep too much, sleep too little)
- fatigue
- preoccupation with death or events surrounding death
- searching for reasons for the loss (sometimes with results that make no sense to others)
- dwelling on mistakes, real or imagined, that you made with the deceased
- guilt
- feeling all alone and distant
- global feeling of anger
- global feeling of envy

Bereavement Counseling

The grieving process can be very painful and difficult for people who have lost someone close to them. Bereavement counseling is a special type of professional help. You may be able to find it through your health insurance, community mental health resources, or hospice programs.

Emotional support can make all the difference in how you recover from your loss and in how much time it takes you to accept your loss. As a grieving person, you need emotional support. Sources of this emotional support can be your family and friends, members of the community, or mental health professionals.

Accepting the Loss

As you begin to slowly accept the loss of your loved one, you are realizing what it means to live without them. You have felt the pain and grief of being without your loved one in your day-to-day life. This is a slow and lonely process, but you can do it. And this is how you accomplish this process of acceptance, by living one day at a time without your loved one.

Acceptance does not happen overnight. This part of the process is as important as the first stages, and it is not uncommon for someone to spend a year or longer to resolve this emotional conflict. While you may feel the pain subside at times, you may also feel your attachment to your loved one become stronger at times. You may feel emotionally attached to your loved one for years after their death. In time, however, you will be able to separate your emotional energy and accept your loved one's death, and move on with your life in a healthy way.

The Rituals of Mourning

Funerals and community rituals are important parts of letting go of a loved one. The ritual of burial provides closure to your loved one's life, and it also provides an opportunity for a public commitment for you to end your living relationship with them.

Seeing friends and family, preparing for the funeral, and burial often provides structure at this time for the bereaved.

Grieving Can Go On for Many Years

After acceptance, more loss may occur after the loss of someone who was close to you. If you had future plans with this person, then there will be many future losses to grieve as a result of losing your loved one. This must also be mourned, and this can continue for decades, if not the rest of your life. For example, if you lose a spouse, you may remember this spouse every time you look at your child, and, of course, during what would have been your anniversary or when the spouse would have had their birthday.

Caring for Yourself after Losing Your Loved One

Self-care is a critical factor in caregiving, and this is an important time for self-care. It might be helpful to talk with friends or family members, spend time in your garden, write in your journal, spend time with your children, exercise, read a good book, go to a concert or a movie, cook, or go out for a meal. Whatever you find relaxing or enjoyable, take some time and do this for yourself.

Your life will have changed forever from the day your loved one received the diagnosis of dementia. And for some time, this will be a taxing and painful change, but this will not always be the case. With time, you will be able to return to the happy and fulfilling life you had before. This does not mean you need to forget about your loved one but rather try to make meaning of the life you had together, including the end of your loved one's life. Joining a caregiver's support group can provide you with a meaningful experience of sharing what you have been through with others who are going through a similar experience and you may be able to help. Additionally, knowing others have been through similar experiences that you have been through can help you feel less along in your suffering and can promote healing.

You can make a scrapbook of mementos that remind you of times you spent with your loved one. Use keepsakes that were a part of your loved one's life. Invite other family members to contribute articles a s well and create a family air loom for everyone to enjoy.

12. Burnout, Compassion Fatigue, and Vicarious Trauma

People who help others put themselves at risk for many traumatic experiences even though they themselves are not experiencing the trauma directly. These challenges can be harmful to everybody who helps, whether they are professional caregivers or family members taking care of a loved one. Just by witnessing harm to others, we can be profoundly affected, even traumatized, which is called compassion fatigue and burnout.

Burnout and Compassion Fatigue

When caregivers experience compassion fatigue or burnout, they may have once been enthusiastic and passionate about the way in which they provided care for others. But they may begin to feel tired and withdrawn or numb and frustrated about helping others. This may lead them to isolate and feel alone and perhaps even angry toward those they help. The need to reach out and help is still there, but it is complicated with a personal sense of reduced motivation, low energy, and an overwhelming sense of hopelessness.

Burnout and *compassion fatigue* are labels used to describe a constellation of symptoms of emotional depletion and a loss of motivation and inability to continue to commit to our caregiving. It is an idiosyncratic symptom-set that includes exhaustion, depersonalization of people we help, and a sense of a lack of personal accomplishment. Emotional exhaustion includes feelings of being overextended, hopeless, and helpless. Depersonalization describes a negative, or callous, response to other people with an inability to attach in a meaningful way. Lack of personal accomplishment refers to a decline in our feeling of competence and successful achievement in our caregiving. Specific symptoms of burnout and compassion fatigue can include depression, cynicism, detachment, loss of vitality, insomnia, loss of intimacy (social and sexual), impatience, anger at people we help, many somatic symptoms (including tension and headaches), susceptibility to illness, apathy, substance abuse, self-harm, decreased productivity, absenteeism, and a decrease in the quality of our caregiving.

Burnout and compassion fatigue often follow a distinct pattern. In the beginning, the caregiver might over identify with the client or loved one and may feel excessively enthusiastic. Then the caregiver becomes overoptimistic and hopeful regarding the client's prognosis. Soon the caregiver moves toward stagnation and disappointment around caregiving expectations sets in. As our caregiving expectations slowly begin to move toward a more realistic place, we can become dissatisfied and personally frustrated. When frustration and anger occurs, a sense of discouragement may cause us to withdraw and isolate from the loved one or client. Finally, we may begin to feel depressed and apathetic and may remove ourselves from the caregiving situation.

Personal or individual characteristics can also influence the onset and severity of this condition with helpers. Those with high self-esteem, or confident individuals, can minimize the external risk factors by possessing what we call resilience.

There are also characteristics about individual personalities and the way in which different individuals "help" that can affect how or if compassion fatigue manifests. Helpers who define most of their identity *as* a "helper" put themselves at risk for not asking for help and support for themselves when they most need it. Caregivers' beliefs, attitudes, and behavior also affect the likelihood of burnout. If we need to make the client or loved one feel better, isolate ourselves from other caregivers, overidentify with the loved one or client, expect to receive gestures of gratitude from clients or loved ones, set exceptionally high goals for our loved ones or clients, or possess perfectionist tendencies, we are more likely to experience compassion fatigue.

Vicarious or Secondary Trauma

Vicarious or secondary trauma is a similar experience to compassion fatigue, but can be experienced just by witnessing someone else's trauma. It is different from post-traumatic stress disorder (PTSD) in that PTSD afflicts the person who directly experiences the trauma. Vicarious or secondary trauma disrupts helpers' self-protective beliefs about safety, control, and predictability in the world, and can leave us feeling helpless and hopeless and despairing.

PTSD can be diagnosed when an individual experiences a traumatic event and reacts with intense fear, helplessness, or horror, and develops symptoms that last for at least a month. The symptoms of PTSD include recurrent and intrusive thoughts or flashbacks of the event (such as dreams or feelings that the event was recurring) and intense psychological distress at exposure to symbolic or similar stimuli of the traumatic event. Other symptoms can include avoidance of any stimuli that reminds the person of the traumatic event; increased arousal such as insomnia; poor concentration or memory; and hypervigilance or an exaggerated startle response. Other problems that often co-occur with PTSD are substance abuse, depression, somatic disorders, adjustment disorders, and sleep disturbances (DSM-TR IV, 1998).

Helpers do not necessarily need to witness these traumatic events that occur in their client's or loved one's lives to experience vicarious or secondary trauma. When engaging people who are suffering in this way, vicarious or secondary trauma is a normal response to working with people who have been traumatized themselves.

Not all helpers will become traumatized by their work with traumatized individuals; however some will experience lasting changes in how they see and feel the world around them, which will negatively impact their emotions, relationships, and life in general. The harm caused by these changes depends on what support and treatment the helper receives (just as the people they help) in processing their traumatic experience, whether the trauma is direct or vicarious.

Helpful processing includes self-care for the helper, a strong social support, eating healthy, having outside interests that you enjoy, and having someone to talk to about your concerns. The helper must be able to explore his own personal beliefs that most people hold as true: a belief in personal invulnerability, the perception of the world and life as being meaningful and understandable, and the view of the "self" in a positive way. Traumatic events directly confront some or all of these beliefs, and, until the helper is able to work through their own ambiguity about these beliefs, the same conflicts will continue to emerge with each personal life crisis.

Signs and Symptoms

Caregiver burnout, compassion fatigue, and vicarious or secondary trauma are some things you may not notice, but people you know may notice changes in you and express their concern.

12. Burnout, Compassion

Here are some signs of caregiver burnout, compassion fatigue, and vicarious and secondary trauma:

- being on the verge of tears or crying a lot
- feeling helpless or hopeless
- overreacting to minor annoyances
- feeling constantly tired
- losing interest in work and caregiving
- losing the ability to enjoy pleasurable activities
- decrease in productivity of work
- withdrawing from social contacts
- increasing use of alcohol or stimulants
- nervous habits such as chain smoking
- change in eating patterns
- change in sleeping patterns
- increasing use of medications for sleeplessness, anxiety, depression
- Inability to relax
- Inability to concentrate
- feeling resentful toward those we help
- being frequently short-tempered
- frequent thoughts of death

As a caregiver, you may have many demands on your time, but it is important to allow yourself time for self-care in order to avoid burnout, compassion fatigue, vicarious trauma, and secondary trauma. Self-care practices include anything you enjoy doing and anything that is part of a healthy lifestyle: these practices will be discussed in detail in the following chapter.

Sample Forms

Medication List

Date _____

Patient Name _____

Patient Address _____

Insurance Information _____

_____

_____

_____

_____

_____

_____

Emergency Contact Information _____

_____

_____

Primary Care Physician _____

_____

_____

Contact Information _____

_____

_____

_____

_____

_____

Medications: _____

_____

_____

_____

_____

Contact List

Date _____

Patient Name _____

Patient Address _____

Emergency Contact Information _____

_____

_____

Name _____ Relationship _____

Phone Number_____

Name _____ Relationship _____

Phone Number_____

Name _____ Relationship _____

Phone Number_____

Name _____ Relationship _____

Phone Number_____

Family Members: _____

_____

_____

_____

_____

Friends: _____

_____

_____

_____

_____

_____

Monthly/Quarterly Budget

Income Sources _____

_____

_____

_____

_____

Bank Accounts _____

_____

_____

_____

_____

Other Financial Institutions _____

_____

_____

_____

_____

_____

Health Insurance Carrier/Policy Number _____

_____

_____

_____

_____

_____

12. Burnout, Compassion

Individual Health care Providers _____

_____

_____

_____

_____

_____

Monthly/Quarterly Household Bills _____

_____

_____

_____

_____

_____

Resources
General

Alzheimer's Association

Alzheimer's Association is an organization where professionals, caregivers, family members, and patients can find current research and education regarding Alzheimer's disease. The site includes access to message boards, weekly newsletters, and an Alzheimer's blog. www.alz.org 800-272-3900

Alzheimer's Disease Education and Referral Center

Alzheimer's Disease Education and Referral Center is an organization that offers information about open clinical research trials regarding Alzheimer's disease and related disorders as well as current research findings. www.nia.nih.gov/alzhe 800-438-4380

Alzheimer's Foundation of America

Alzheimer's Foundation of America is a membership community offering support, education, and current research conclusions to family members and caregivers for people with Alzheimer's disease and other dementias. alzfdn.org 866-232-8484

Alzheimer's Store

The Alzheimer's Store is dedicated to providing unique products and information for those caring for someone with Alzheimer's disease. Every product in the store has been carefully selected to make living with Alzheimer's disease as easy as possible. 800-752-3238 www.alzstore.com

ALZTalk

Sponsored by the Fisher Center Foundation, Alztalk is an online community that allows people to stay connected with a safe environment for families, friends, and medical professionals to post messages, pictures, and favorite links. www.alztalk.org

American Association of Poison Control Centers

The American Association of Poison Control Web site offers education regarding poison prevention, patient management, and poison data as wells as news and events surrounding poison control nationwide. There is also a twenty-four-hour hotline to ask questions regarding poisoning possibilities in the home. www.aapcc.org 800-222-1222

Association for Frontotemperal Degeneration

The Association for Frontotemporal Degeneration Web site offers links to open clinical research trials, conferences, and community support for caregivers and family members of patients with frontotemporal dementia and related disorders. www.theaftd.com 866-507-7222

Brightstar

Brightstar is a national full-service agency providing in-home services as well as child-care, respite care, and trained medical staffing. www.brightstarcare.com 877-689-6898

Compare Health Care

Compare Health Care is a Web site that provides information to assist in making informed decisions regarding choosing doctors, hospitals, skilled-nursing facilities, and other resources for loved ones with dementia. www.comparehealthcare.com

Dementia Guide

The Dementia Guide Web site offers education about Alzheimer's disease and related dementias as well as symptoms and phases of dementia. This Web site also has a symptom tracker to follow the progression of the patient's disease. www.dementiaguide.com

Dolls for Alzheimers

Dolls for Alzheimers is an organization that provides (for a fee) therapeutic lifelike dolls for people with dementia. www.dolls4alzheimers.com

Elder Helpline from AARP

Elder Helpline from AARP offers information regarding assisted living communities, legal services, affordable housing, healthcare services, telecommunication services, and other resources. www.elderhelpline.org

Family Care Navigator

Family Care Navigator is a Web site that lists resources state by state, such as government resources, nonprofits, private organizations, and disease-specific organizations. www.familycaregivernavigator.org

Family Caregiver Alliance

Family Caregiver Alliance is part of the National Center on Caregiving and offers support and education through advocacy and training programs. www.familycaregiveralliance.org 800-445-8106

Home Helpers

Home Helpers is a national full-service agency providing home care to individuals with dementia and related disorders as well as respite care and child-care. www.homehelpers.cc 800-216-4196

Hospital Ranking Tool

Hospital Ranking Tool is provided by Consumer Reports as a free online feature that rates major US hospitals on how conservatively or aggressively they treat the top nine causes of death, including dementia. www.consumerreports.org/health/doctors-and-hospital-home.htm

Joint Commission

The Joint Commission provides information regarding health-care organization's accreditation and certification standards as wells as national performance rankings of health-care organizations. www.jointcommission.org 630-792-5800

Know It Alz

Offering humor and help with seeing the brighter side of caregiving, Know It Alz is a daily blog for caregivers of people with dementia. www.knowitalz.com

Law Depot

Law Depot offers free, do-it-yourself online preparation of many legal documents like wills, durable power of attorney, and advanced health care directives. www.lawdepot.com

Law Office of Christopher M. Guest, PLLC

Estate Planning, Probate & Trust Administration, General Business Advice

866 16th Street, NW, Suite 800

Washington, DC 20006
202-349-3969
Arlington, VA 22207
703-574-5654
cguest@guestlawllc.com

Legal Zoom

Legal Zoom offers online legal preparation of many different legal documents like wills, durable power of attorney, and advanced health care directives. www.legalzoom.com

Lewy Body Dementia Association

Lewy Body Dementia Association is an organization where family members, caregivers, and professionals can find information about current research, support, information, and treatment facts regarding Lewy Body Dementia. www.lbda.org800-539-9767

McCurdy, Lisa, Esq.

At The Wealth Counselor, LLC, we counsel clients on all aspects of estate planning - wills, trusts, durable powers of attorney, asset-protection, business legacy and succession strategies, planned giving, guardianship and the preservation of government benefits for the elderly and disabled. For business clients, in particular, we identify areas of exposure and establish methods to ensure their assets create a legacy for generations to come. It is especially important for business owners and other dealmakers to protect their personal assets from business transactions, impatient investors and other potentially damaging circumstance that could affect their family's well-being.

Further, as our clients build their team of advisors, we try to offer a "one-stop-shop" referral service through a network of partnerships across disciplines such as insurance, financial management, accounting and tax planning. 202-552-7383 lgmccurdy@ thewealthcounselor.com

MD Junction

Providing support for people dealing with Alzheimer's disease and other dementias, MD Junction is an online community to trade stories and "hugs" and offer support to other group members. There is also an option to ask a physician questions online. wwwmdjunction.com

Medicare

Medicare is the federal health insurance program that covers most people age sixty-five and older. 800-633-4227

Memory Jogging Puzzles

Memory Jogging Puzzles is a company that offers puzzles and card games designed to benefit those with memory loss and their families.www.memoryjoggingpuzzles.com

Missingpatient.com

Missingpatient.com is a company that offers software and a corresponding call center as a comprehensive solution for patients who wander and subsequently may become lost or missing. www.missingpatient.com

National Association to Stop Guardian Abuse

National Association to Stop Guardian Abuse is an organization that advocates against conservatorship laws to protect people from guardian/conservatorship abuse. www.stopguardianabuse.org

National Alliance for Caregiving

National Alliance for Caregiving is an organization where caregivers and family members can find information about current research findings and resources for education about dementia. www.caregiving.org

National Crisis Support Hotline

National Crisis Support Hotline provides suicide prevention, intervention, and aftercare services as well as providing local community resources for crisis intervention. 800-273-8255

National Institute on Aging

National Institute on Aging offers this Web site to provide links for information about open clinical research trials as well as current research findings and resources for professionals. www.nih.gov

National Pet Loss Helpline (ASPCA)

ASPCA National Pet Loss Helpline offers free nationwide consultation to bereaved animal owners on a twenty-four-hour basis. www.griefhealing.com 877-474-3310

National Suicide Prevention Lifeline

National Suicide Prevention Lifeline is free, twenty-four-hour crisis support for anyone who is experiencing emotional stress. 800-273-8255 www.suicidepreventionlifeline.org

Senior Decision

Senior Decision is a Web site that features consumer ratings and reviews regarding senior care and senior housing.www.seniordecision.com

Appendix A

Euthanasia Organizations

Exit International

Exit International is a leading end-of-life-choices information and advocacy organization, founded by Philip Nitschke, PhD, MD. Exit International holds regular meetings in the UK, Ireland, Australia, North America, and New Zealand. Exit was previously known as the Voluntary Euthanasia Research Foundation.   www.exitinternational.net

Euthanasia Research & Guidance Organization (ERGO)

ERGO's mission is to provide information and literature on the right to choose to die by a competent adult, either by assisted suicide or self-deliverance. ERGO, incorporated under Oregon law in 1993 as a nonprofit educational organization, has more than five thousand supporters. ERGO maintains three Web sites—www.finalexit.org, www.assistedsuicide.org, and www.assistedsuicide.org/blog—and delivers an Internet news digest, focusing on right-to-die issues, to subscribers around the world. ERGO's bookstore distributes Final Exit, the well-known "how-to" book by Derek Humphry, and contributes the profits to other right-to-die groups. Since 1999, ERGO has hosted the suicide device research group NuTech, which meets in various world cities to examine new ways of legal self-deliverance.

Death with Dignity National Center

The mission of the Death with Dignity National Center is to provide information, education, research, and support for the preservation, implementation, and promotion of Death with Dignity laws, which allow a terminally ill, mentally competent adult the right to request and receive a prescription to hasten death under certain specific safeguards. This organization promotes Death with Dignity laws based on Oregon's model legislation, the Oregon Death with Dignity Act, as a stimulus to nationwide improvements in end-of-life care and as an option for dying individuals. This organization accomplishes this mission by working to defend and promote Death with Dignity laws in court and in the court of public opinion.   www.deathwithdignity.org

Compassion & Choices

Once known as the Hemlock Society, Compassion & Choices is a non-profit organization that provides education to anyone interested in options regarding health care and end-of-life choices. Part of the mission includes educating the public about why people suffering from end-of-life issues might want to end terminal suffering premature to their natural death. Compassion & Choices has been active in the legislative process in trying to pass laws to help give terminally ill and mentally able patients a choice in their end-of-life options.   www.compassionandchoices.org

Final Exit Network

Final Exit Network is a nonprofit organization that is run by volunteers. It is one of the newer organizations in support of assisted suicide as it has been in operation only for the past four years. The four goals of their mission statement are: to offer free service to all who apply, providing relevant information, home visits if possible, and compassionate counseling for individual and family; to raise the awareness of all Americans concerning this basic human right; to promote the use of advance directives and other related legal instruments; to document the intentions of any individual; to sponsor research into new peaceful and reliable methods to end life; and to vigorously defend our guiding principle in a court of law when necessary.   www.finalexitnetwork.org

Dignity in Dying

Dignity in Dying is a voluntary organization located in London. Organized by volunteers, they campaign for a change in the law on assisted dying for terminally ill and mentally competent adults. They do this by lobbying decision-makers, educating legal and healthcare professionals, and empowering terminally ill people and their loved ones, who are suffering under the current system, to have their voices heard. Alongside their campaigning, Compassion in Dying undertakes research on end-of-life care, provides free advance decisions, and works to educate and empower people around their existing rights at the end of life.   www.dignityindying.org

Dying with Dignity Victoria

Dying with Dignity is based in Canada and strives to improve dying individuals' quality of dying and expand Canadians' end-of-life choices by providing education about end-of-life options and the importance of advance care planning; support for individuals at the end of their lives, including support at the bedside of those who wish to determine the nature and timing of their death; and information about the choice in dying movement and the reasons why appropriately regulated medically assisted dying should be legalized in Canada.   www.dignitywithdying.ca

Dignity New Zealand

It is the belief of this organization that terminally ill patients should have the option of assisted suicide and should not be punished if opting to do so. The parliament of New Zealand has rejected two pieces of legislation regarding the use of assisted suicide for terminally ill patients. Although both of these attempts were upsetting for the Dignity NZ organization, they are continuing with their agenda to make assisted suicide for terminally ill patients a viable choice. The members of this organization understand that freedom of choice is essential for complete human identity and realize that free choices should also be incorporated with death and dying decisions.   www.dignity.co.nz

The World Federation of Right to Die Societies

The World Federation, founded in 1980, consists of forty-five right to die organizations from twenty-six countries. The Federation provides an international link for organizations working to secure or protect the rights of individuals to self-determination at the end of their lives. The Federation disseminates current information and educational materials about voluntary euthanasia, physician-assisted dying, other right-to-die issues, and related matters of interest; promotes cooperation and liaison among our member societies; facilitates international conferences on dying and death; provides assistance, where requested, to groups and individuals interested in establishing similar societies in countries where such societies do not currently exist; and responds to requests by interested groups, scholars, and individuals for information about right-to-die issues.

The World Federation of Right to Die Societies summarizes its views in a manifesto. They meet every two years to exchange news and views, to elect directors and officers of the Federation, and to conduct other business.   www.worldrtd.net

Euthanasia Literature

Final Exit: The Practicalities of Self-Deliverance and Assisted Suicide for the Dying

by Derek Humphry   ISBN 978-0-9637280-6-7

Final Exit is perhaps one of the most popular texts on the topic of assisted suicide and euthanasia. Includes unique plain and simple language for a competent adult who is terminally and wishing to bring their life to a peaceful, nonviolent end. This can be achieved without permission or assistance of any doctor. For example, drug dosages and helium gas techniques are described and illustrated as well as suggestions given about where and how to obtain supplies to carry out such techniques.

Final Exit describes similar methods that are used by Dignitas (Switzerland) and other right-to-die groups in the Netherlands, Belgium, Luxembourg, Colombia, and countries where euthanasia laws have been passed. Final Exit also outlines the legal complications connected with dying, death, hastened death, euthanasia laws, suicide, living wills, and advance directives. Issues like who the person should tell about their plans and the advisability of a "suicide note" are also addressed. The problems with life insurance are clarified. The difficult issues of double suicide and hastened death for persons with disabilities are also frankly discussed.

Appendices references include a glossary of terms connected with dying; alternative euphemistic terms for assisted dying and death; International and US right-to-die law, including the Oregon Death with Dignity Act, etc.

The Good Euthanasia Guide: Where, What, and Who in Choices in Dying
by Derek Humphry   ISBN 978-0-97683283-1-0

The Good Euthanasia Guide provides vital information about assisted suicide and euthanasia. This desk reference includes several chapters dealing with the future of the right-to-die movement. All the world's organizations are listed, as well as a summary of international laws, a filmography, and a bibliography. It also contains an analysis of the work of Dr. Jack Kevorkian. This is not a how-to book like Final Exit but a guidebook to euthanasia in general, worldwide. It discusses places where euthanasia is legal and where it is not. It discusses where to find Dignitas in Switzerland, where is the Hemlock Society still operating, what about Dutch euthanasia, and so forth.

Let Me Die Before I Wake
by Derek Humphry   ISBN 0-440-50477-5

This book contains the true stories of persons dying of a terminal or hopeless illness and how they achieved their desired assisted death. It was written by journalist and author Derek Humphry ten years before his famous "how-to" bestseller Final Exit; nevertheless, Let Me Die contains crucial drug, technical, and personal information needed for successful euthanasia. Let Me Die was the main publication of the original Hemlock Society and has helped thousands to achieve the right to die in peace and dignity. It has been factually updated and extended over time in new editions.

Jean's Way: A Love Story

by Derek Humphry   ISBN 0963728075

This book is a moving account by a terminally ill woman's husband of her carefully planned self-deliverance, with his help, from suffering. An international bestseller in five languages since 1978, now considered a classic in the euthanasia field, this book led to the founding of the Hemlock Society USA in 1980 and the passage of the Oregon Death with Dignity Act in 1994.

Euthanasia Weblog

Euthanasia, Assisted Suicide, Right-to-Die, Final Exit, Hemlock Society Founder Weblog

This Web site is a Weblog where up-to-date information is posted regarding assisted suicide and euthanasia. Information about local and international organizations can be found as well as current legislation and how to get involved with advocating for change in legislation. Derek Humphry, the author of the three books on euthanasia listed above, runs this Weblog.   www.self-deliverance.blogspot.com

Author Bio

Dr. Francis has resided in Northern California since the early 1980's where she attended Mills College and John F. Kennedy University earning a doctoral degree in clinical psychology. As part of her doctoral studies, Dr. Francis conducted original research on arranged marriage for her dissertation. Currently, as a clinical psychologist, Dr. Francis treats patients for a variety of psychiatric conditions, including dementia and related disorders.

Dr. Francis has significant experience working with the geriatric population. Prior to graduate school, she worked with hospice patients and provided end-of-life treatments for both patients and family members. During graduate school, Dr. Francis provided psychotherapy for geriatric patients by way of home-visits as well as telephone counseling to ensure inclusion of all people, not only those who could travel to office settings.

Currently, Dr. Francis enjoys writing about topics of interest to older adults because she is interested is sharing her knowledge with the population with which she has had the most experience. Other topics Dr. Francis has written about include sexuality and euthanasia rights for terminally ill patients.

References

Alzheimer's Association. 2012. <www.alz.org>

Alzheimer's Disease Education. 2012. <www.nia.nih.gov/alzhe>

Alzheimer's Foundation of America. 2011. <www.alzfdn.org>

Alzheimer's Store. 2011. <www.alzdtore.com>

alztalk. 2012. <www.alztalk.org>

American Association of Poison Control. 2012. <www.aapcc.org>

Association for Frontotemperal Dementia. 2011. <www.theaftd.com>

Brightstar. 2011. <www.brightstarcare.com

Compare Health Care. 2011. <www.comparehealthcare.com>

Compassion & Choices. 2010. <www.compassionandchoices.org>

Death with Dignity National Center. 2010. <www.deathwithdignity.org>

Dementia Guide. 2011. <www.dementiahealthguide.com>

Dolls for Alzheimer's. 2011. <www.dolls4alzheimers.com>

Dying with Dignity. 2010. <www.dignityindying.org>

Elder Helpline from AARP. 2011. <www.elderhelpline.org>

Exit International. 2010. <www.exitinternational.net>

Family Care Navigator. 2012. <www.familycaregivernavigator.org>

Family Caregiver Alliance. 2010. <www.familycaregiveralliance.org>

Home Helpers. 2011. <www.homehelpers.cc>

Hospital Ranking Tool. 2010. <www.consumerreports.org>

Joint Commission. 2010. <www.jointcommission.org>

Know it Alz. 2011. <www.knowitalz.com>

Law Depot. 2011. <www.lawdepot.com>

Guest, C., M., Esq. 2012. <cguest@guestlawllc.com>

Legal Zoom. 2011. <www.legalzoom.com>

Lewy Body Dementia Association. 2010. <www.lbda.com>

Mayo Clinic. 2010. <www.mayoclinic.com>

McCurdy, L., Esq. (2012). Advanced Health Care Directive. lmccurdy@thewealthcounselor.com

(reprinted with permission of the copyright holder: Mccurdy, L.)

McCurdy, L., Esq. (2012). Durable Power of Attorney. lgmccurdy@thewealthcounselor.com

(reprinted with permission of the copyright holder: Mccurdy, L.)

McCurdy, L., Esq. (2012). Living Will and Trust. lgmccurdy@thewealthcounselor.com

(reprinted with permission of the copyright holder: Mccurdy, L.)

MD Junction. 2011. <www.mdjunction.com>

Medicare. 2010. <www.medicare,gov>

Memory Jogging Puzzles. 2012. <www.memoryjoggingpuzzles.com>

Missing patient.com. 2010. <www.missingpatientcom>

National Association to Stop Guardian Abuse. 2010. <www.stopguardianabuse.org>

National Alliance for Caregiving. 2012. <www.caregiving.org>

National Institute on Aging. 2011. <www.nih.gov>

National Pet Loss Helpline, 2011. (ASPCA) <www.griefline.com>

National Suicide Prevention Lifeline. 2010. <www.suicidepreventionlifeline.org>

Senior Decision. 2011. <www.seniordecision.com>